Rad Tech's Guide to
MRI: Imaging Procedures, Patient Care, and Safety

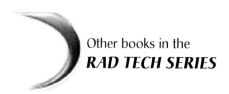

Other books in the
RAD TECH SERIES

Rad Tech's Guide to MRI: Imaging Procedures, Patient Care, and Safety

Carolyn Kaut Roth, RT(R), (MR), (CT), (M), (CV)
Director Technologist Continuing Education
and MRI Programs
University of Pennsylvania Medical Center
Philadelphia, Pennsylvania

Series Editor
Euclid Seeram, RTR, BSc, MSc, FCAMRT
Medical Imaging Advanced Studies
British Columbia Institute of Technology
Burnaby, British Columbia, Canada

b
**Blackwell
Science**

EDITORIAL OFFICES:
Commerce Place, 350 Main Street, Malden, Massachusetts 02148, USA
Osney Mead, Oxford OX2 0EL, England
25 John Street, London WC1N 2BS, England
23 Ainslie Place, Edinburgh EH3 6AJ, Scotland
54 University Street, Carlton, Victoria 3053, Australia

OTHER EDITORIAL OFFICES:
Blackwell Wissenschafts-Verlag GmbH, Kurfürstendamm 57, 10707 Berlin, Germany
Blackwell Science KK, MG Kodenmacho Building, 7-10 Kodenmacho Nihombashi,
    Chuo-ku, Tokyo 104, Japan
Iowa State University Press, A Blackwell Science Company, 2121 S. State Avenue,
    Ames, Iowa 50014-8300, USA

DISTRIBUTORS:
The Americas
  Blackwell Publishing
  c/o AIDC
  P.O. Box 20
  50 Winter Sport Lane
  Williston, VT 05495-0020
  (Telephone orders: 800-216-2522;
      fax orders: 802-864-7626)
Australia
  Blackwell Science Pty, Ltd.
  54 University Street
  Carlton, Victoria 3053
  (Telephone orders: 03-9347-0300;
      fax orders: 03-9349-3016)

Outside The Americas and Australia
  Blackwell Science, Ltd.
  c/o Marston Book Services, Ltd.
  P.O. Box 269
  Abingdon
  Oxon OX14 4YN
  England
  (Telephone orders: 44-01235-465500;
      fax orders: 44-01235-465555)

Acquisitions: Beverly Copland
Development: Julia Casson
Production: GraphCom Corporation
Manufacturing: Lisa Flanagan
Marketing Manager: Toni Fournier
Cover and interior design: Dana Peick, GraphCom Corporation
Typesetting: GraphCom Corporation

Printed in the United States of America
    7   2008

The Blackwell Science logo is a trade mark of Blackwell Science Ltd., registered
at the United Kingdom Trade Marks Registry.

Library of Congress Cataloging-in-Publication Data

Kaut Roth, Carolyn.
    Rad tech's guide to MRI : imaging procedures, patient care, and safety / by
Carolyn Kaut Roth.
        p. ; cm.
    ISBN 978-0-632-04507-5
    1. Magnetic resonance imaging—Outlines, syllabi, etc. 2. Radiologic technolo-
gists—Outlines, syllabi, etc. I. Title: Guide to MRI. II. Title.
    [DNLM: 1. Magnetic Resonance Imaging—methods—Outlines. 2. Technology,
Radiologic—methods—Outlines. WN 18.2 K21ra2001]
    RC78.7.N83 K386 2001
    616.07'548—dc21
                                                      2001025055

TABLE OF CONTENTS

SERIES EDITOR'S FOREWORD

Blackwell Science's Rad Tech Series in radiologic technology is intended to provide a clear and comprehensive coverage of a wide range of topics and prepare students to write their entry-to-practice registration examination. Additionally, this series can be used by working technologists to review essential and practical concepts and principles and to use them as tools to enhance their daily skills during the examination of patients in the radiology department.

The Rad Tech Series features short books covering the fundamental core curriculum topics for radiologic technologists at both the diploma and the specialty levels, as well as act as knowledge sources for continuing education as defined by the American Registry for Radiologic Technologists (ARRT).

The entry-to-practice series includes books on radiologic physics, equipment operation, patient care, radiographic technique, radiologic procedures, radiation protection, image production and evaluation, and quality control. This specialty series features books on computed tomography physics and instrumentation, patient care and safety, and imaging procedures; mammography; and quality management in imaging sciences.

In *Rad Tech's Guide to MRI: Imaging Procedures, Patient Care, and Safety,* Carolyn Kaut Roth, a renowned educator and director technologist of MR programs of the University of Pennsylvania Medical Center, presents clear and concise coverage of patient care and safety issues of magnetic resonance imaging (MRI), as well as MR imaging procedures. Topics include patient care and safety, imaging procedures that describe MRI of the head and neck, spine, chest, musculoskeletal system abdomen, pelvis, and vascular system.

Carolyn Kaut Roth has done an excellent job in explaining significant concepts that are mandatory for the successful per-

formance of quality MRI in clinical practice. Students, technologists, and educators alike will find this book a worthwhile
addition to their libraries.

Enjoy the pages that follow; remember, your patients will
benefit from your wisdom.

Euclid Seeram, RTR, BSc, MSc, FCAMRT
Series Editor
British Columbia, Canada

PREFACE

The purpose of *Rad Tech's Guide to MRI: Imaging Procedures, Patient Care, and Safety* is to provide an easy reference for the study of magnetic resonance imaging (MRI) for the technologist who is preparing for the advanced level examination in MRI. This guide can also be used as a quick overview of MRI for the practicing technologist and physician. The outline format provides easy reference for each section of the text. The subtopics and bulleted text facilitate quick reference without "over reading" the material.

MRI safety and imaging procedures with anatomy have been discussed in this guide, and the basic principles and image contrast to pulse sequences and k-space are discussed in a partner guide in the Rad Tech series. The more complicated topics have hopefully been expressed in an understandable format that will encourage the reader to explore these topics, rather than run in the opposite direction. Purists may perceive our attempt at creating a "user-friendly" text as an oversimplification. However, we believe it important to disseminate difficult information to a variety of educational levels.

Carolyn Kaut Roth

ACKNOWLEDGMENTS

First, I would like to thank God for the opportunity to be involved in this project, the wisdom to undertake it, and the determination to see it through.

Next, I gratefully acknowledge the encouragement of those individuals who have given me the support and patience to complete this guide. These include my loving husband, Scott, and the rest of my family—my mom, dad, brothers, in-laws, nieces, and nephews. I love you all.

My thanks, however, cannot end with my family. My extended "HUP" family was also instrumental in providing information and images for the text. In particular, I would like to thank Lisa Desiderio, Paula Malagoli, Tony Festa, Dave Flint, Jorge Forero, Camille Gallen, Christy Lennen, Joe Shea, Lena Inverso, Doree Schrann, Russell Boucher, Lee Cohen, Doris Caine-Edwards, Beverly Farrar, Nancy Fedullo, Jim Garrisson, Christine Harris, Dave Yost, Mike Irvin, Ralph Magee, Ray Chemiewlewslki, Ted Czwoski, and Ann Kopp, my office mate. Without your support, this project would have been virtually impossible.

—CKR

CHAPTER 1

Patient Care and Safety for Magnetic Resonance Imaging

Chapter at a glance

INTRODUCTION TO PATIENT CARE AND SAFETY FOR MRI

To date, there have been virtually no long-term adverse biologic effects of extended exposure to magnetic resonance imaging (MRI) in general. However, when separate components of the MRI process are examined, several inconsequential and reversible effects of magnetic, gradient, and radio frequency (RF) fields can be observed. When MRI systems began to be used in the United States, the Food and Drug Administration (FDA) issued guidelines to hospital's Investigational Review Boards (IRBs) in "Guidelines for Evaluating Electromagnetic Exposure Risks for Trials of Clinical NMR Systems," on February 25, 1982. Follow-up was presented in December of that same year, not intending to provide limitations, but rather to evaluate the need for a risk assessment. Therefore the need to evaluate MRI for potential risks and hazards is clear and, to validly discuss long-term biologic effects of MRI, all of the components of the imaging process should be considered. These elements include not only the main magnetic field known as the static magnetic field (B_0), but also time-varying magnetic fields caused by magnetic field gradients and RF fields (B_1) created by RF transmitters and receiver coils.

The purpose of this chapter is to explore the safety aspects of MRI.

SCREENING PATIENTS AND PERSONNEL

Conducting a careful screening procedure is crucial to ensure the safety of anyone who enters the area of the magnetic resonance (MR) system. Careful questioning and education of patients and personnel help to maintain this controlled environment. Patient and personnel screening is, to date, the most effective way to avoid potential health hazards to patients involved in MRI. Patients and MR personnel with questionable ferromagnetic foreign objects either in or on their bodies should be rigorously examined so as to avoid any serious health risks or accidents.

- All individuals, including patients, volunteer subjects, visitors, MR health care providers, and custodial workers, must be thoroughly screened by qualified personnel before being exposed to the MRI environment. In addition, routine preventative maintenance checks by the service engineer, as well as continuing education is also important. Therefore careful planning and diligent upkeep of the MR facility can provide a safe environment for patients, visitors, and employees.

- Most MR-related injuries have been a direct result of deficiencies in screening methods. Unfortunately, not all MR users perform a rigorous screening procedure and there is a lack of agreement on what constitutes an appropriate or necessary protocol that will ensure the safety of individuals and patients in the MR setting. One other note is warranted: *If a patient has previously had an MR examination, this is not an indication that they are safe to undergo another.*

In 1994 the safety committee of the International Society for Magnetic Resonance in Medicine (previously designated as the Society for Magnetic Resonance Imaging) published screening recommendations and a questionnaire that encompassed all of the important aforementioned issues. These recommendations were developed from a consensus from an international panel of MR experts and were intended for use as a standard of care at all MR centers. Elster and others (1994) also published a screening recommendation. This information was somewhat similar to the content of the recommendations provided by the safety committee, which is not surprising since many of the same MR clinicians and scientists were involved in the development of both documents. A comprehensive pre-MRI screening form may be downloaded from the Internet (Mrsafety.com) and used at MRI facilities. This form was recently developed in collaboration with Frank Shellock and Anne Sawyer-Glover (1999).

Pre-MRI Screening Form or Questionnaire

The initial screening process should involve completion of a questionnaire that is specifically designed to determine whether there is any reason that the individual would have an adverse reaction to the MRI environment.

- The questionnaire must include important questions concerning previous surgery, prior injury from a metallic foreign body, and whether the individual is pregnant.
- In addition, the questionnaire should contain a means of determining whether the individual has any of the various implants, materials, devices, or objects that are considered to be a contraindication or problematic in the MR environment, including any device that is electrically, magnetically, or mechanically activated.
- A diagram of the human body should be provided on the questionnaire for the individual to indicate the position of any object that would be potentially hazardous or would interfere with the interpretation of the MR procedure as a result of causing what is known as an artifact.
- The pre-MRI screening questionnaire may also be used to obtain additional pertinent information related to the safe performance of the MR procedure. For example, questions may be asked concerning previous adverse reactions to contrast media that should alert the health care provider to potential problems.
- Finally, pertinent questions should include information related to the phase of the menstrual cycle, as well as the use of contrast media and hormone treatment that are relevant to patients undergoing MRI examinations for breast abnormalities.

Pre-MRI Screening Interview

With the use of any form of written questionnaire, limitations related to incomplete or incorrect answers provided by the patient, guardian, or other individual preparing to enter the MRI environment are bound to exist. For example, there may be difficulties associated with individuals who are impaired with respect to their vision, fluency, or level of literacy. Therefore it may be necessary to have a version of the screening questionnaire in the individual's native language or to have a direct verbal interaction with individuals who may routinely have problems with written questionnaires.

- It is also recommended that the MR technologist or other trained staff member conduct an oral interview to further ensure the safety of the individual entering the

MRI environment or undergoing an MR procedure. This allows a mechanism for clarification or confirmation of the answers to the questions posed to the individual so that there is no miscommunication.

- The "oral phase" of pre-MRI screening is believed to be especially vital for establishing the reliability of the individual's answer.

Prescreening for Metallic Implants

Every MRI facility must establish a standardized policy for pre-MRI screening of patients and individuals who are suspected of having metallic foreign objects. The policy should include guidelines concerning which individuals or patients require "work-up" by radiographic procedures and the specific procedure to be performed (e.g., number and type of views, position of the anatomy). Each case must be considered on an individual basis to assess the relative risk with regard to the metal object and the MRI environment. These basic precautions should be taken with respect to any type of MR system regardless of the field strength, magnet type, and the presence or absence of magnetic shielding.

Pregnant Patients

A patient who is pregnant or suspects that she is pregnant must be identified before exposure to the MRI environment to address the risks versus the benefits of the examination for the individual. To date, there are no known biologic effects of MRI on fetuses. However, a number of mechanisms exist whereby there could be a potential for adverse effects of the interaction of electromagnetic fields with developing fetuses. Cells undergoing division, which occurs during the first trimester of pregnancy, are more susceptible to a variety of effects. For this reason, many facilities choose to delay MR imaging until after the first trimester.

The FDA guidelines indicate that the safety of MRI when used to image the fetus has not been established or proved. Therefore patients should be provided this information and should also be informed that there are presently no known deleterious effects related to the use of MR procedures during pregnancy. However, according to the recommendations provided by the safety committee of the Society for Magnetic Resonance Imaging, "MR procedures may be used for pregnant patients when other nonionizing forms of diagnostic imaging are inadequate or when the examination provides important information that would otherwise require exposure to a diagnostic procedure that requires ionizing radiation (e.g., computerized tomography, fluoroscopy)." For this reason, the American College of Gynecology and Obstetrics recommends that potential MR patients who are pregnant should be reviewed on a case-by-case basis. This policy has been adopted by the American College of Radiology and is considered to be the "standard of care" with respect to the use of MR procedures for pregnant patients.

Pregnant Employees

A recent survey revealed no increased incidence of spontaneous abortions among MR technologists and health care practitioners. (It should be noted that the incidence of spontaneous abortions makes up approximately 30% of all pregnancies.) After this survey, the following determinations were made:

- The facility from which the data was observed changed their in-house policy from one which restricts pregnant technologists from being near the magnetic field to a policy which allows pregnant technologists to be in the room to set up the patient but not to remain in the room during image acquisition.

- It has been suggested that informed workers make their own decision. For this reason, MRI facilities have established individual guidelines for pregnant employees in the MR environment. The majority of facilities have determined that pregnant employees can safely enter the scan room of superconductors or permanent magnets on which the magnetic field is contained, but must stay out while the scanner is running when the RF and gradient fields are employed.

- A policy is recommended that permits pregnant technologists and health care workers to perform MR procedures, as well as to enter the MR system room and to attend to the patient during pregnancy, regardless of the trimester.

■ Importantly, the technologists or health care worker should not remain in the MR system room or magnet bore during the actual operation of the device. This recommendation is especially important for MR users involved in interventional MR-guided examinations and procedures to which to adhere since it may be necessary for them to be directly exposed to the MR system's electromagnetic fields at levels similar to the fields used for patients. Notably, these recommendations are not based on indications of adverse effects, but rather from a conservative point of view and the notion that there are insufficient data pertaining to the effects of the other electromagnetic fields of the MR system to support or allow unnecessary exposures. This recommendation was influenced by a government legal decision concerning the rights of pregnant workers in hazardous environments.

■ As an additional precaution, some facilities recommend that the employee stay out of the magnetic field entirely during the first trimester of pregnancy.

ANCILLARY EQUIPMENT AND IMPLANTS

To deem ancillary equipment safe for use in MRI, the FDA recommends one of three criteria: manufacturer declaration, FDA approval, and prior testing. Manufacturer declaration simply means that the manufacturer has tested the equipment and assures its safety. FDA approval means that the FDA has tested the material and determined that it is safe for use in MRI. The third requirement means that the instrument has been subjected to *prior testing*, which means that someone has tested the instrument before its use in MRI.

Implants and Prostheses

As we consider metallic implants and their safety profile in the MR environment, three serious effects become clear: torque, heating, and artifactual results on MR images.

Therefore before we consider imaging patients using MR, be aware of surgical procedures that the patient has undergone before the MR examination. For a complete list of MR-compatible implants and prosthesis, refer to "MR Imaging and Biomedical

Implants, Materials, and Devices: An Updated Review" in *Radiology* magazine (1991).

Torque and Heating

Some metallic implants have shown considerable torque when placed in the presence of a magnetic field.

- The force or torque exerted on small and large metallic implants can cause serious effects since unanchored implants have the potential of unpredictable movement within the body.

- The type of metal used in these implants is one factor that determines the force exerted on them in magnetic fields. Although nonferrous, metallic implants may show little or no deflection to the field, they can cause significant heating as a result of their inability to dissipate heat from RF absorption.

Artifacts from Metallic Implants

Although artifacts cannot be considered as biologic effects of the MR process, misinterpretation of MR images can yield devastating consequences. It should be noted that the type of metal and the size of the metallic implant determines the size of the artifact noted on the MR image. Therefore when a metal artifact is noted on the MR image and no metal is present within the patient, the presence of blood products suggestive of a hemorrhagic lesion may be indicated.

The presence of an aneurysm clip in a patient referred for an MR procedure represents a situation that requires the utmost consideration because of the associated risks (Figure 1-1). Certain types of intracranial aneurysm clips (i.e., clips made from martensitic stainless steels, such as 17-7PH or 405 stainless steel) are an absolute contraindication to the use of MR procedures because excessive magnetically induced forces can displace these clips and cause serious injury or death. By comparison, aneurysm clips classified as *nonferromagnetic* or *weakly ferromagnetic* (i.e., those made from Phynox, Elgiloy, austenitic stainless steels, titanium alloy, commercially pure titanium) are safe for patients undergoing MR procedures. For the sake of discussion, the term "weakly ferromagnetic" refers to metal that may demonstrate some extremely low ferromag-

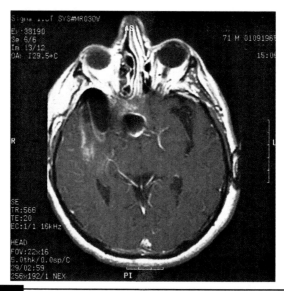

Figure 1-1 This axial image of the brain demonstrates a patient who has had two aneurysm clips implanted. Note that the metal artifacts are different sizes (smaller toward midline and larger toward the right side just behind the orbit), which probably indicates that these clips are made from different trace metals. (Both clips were deemed safe for MRI.)

netic qualities using highly sensitive measurements techniques (e.g., vibrating sample magnetometer, superconducting quantum interference device, SQUID magnetometer), and, as such, may not be technically referred to as being *nonferromagnetic.* It is further recognized that all metals possess some degree of magnetism, such that no metal is considered to be totally *nonmagnetic* or *nonferromagnetic.*

■ It is not uncommon to use MR procedures to evaluate patients with certain types of aneurysm clips. Becker et al, "using MR systems that ranged from 0.35 to 0.60 Tesla (T), studied three patients with nonferromagnetic aneurysm clips (one patient, Yasargil, 316 LVM stainless steel; two patients, Vari-Angle McFadden, MP35N; 316 LVM) and one patient with a ferromagnetic aneurysm clip (Heifetz aneurysm clip, 17-7PH) without incident."

Similarly, Dujovny et al have reported no adverse effects in patients with nonferromagnetic aneurysm clips who have undergone procedures using 1.5 T MR systems.

■ It is therefore recommended that MR imaging in patients with aneurysm clips be delayed until such time that the type of clip is emphatically identified as nonferrous.

Hemostatic Vascular Clips

Hemostatic clips should be evaluated ex vivo before the MR exam, although none of the six hemostatic vascular clips evaluated has shown deflection by the static magnetic field.

■ To date, none of the various hemostatic vascular clips evaluated was attracted by static magnetic fields up to 1.5 T. These hemostatic clips are made from nonferromagnetic materials such as tantalum and nonferromagnetic forms of stainless steel.

■ There has never been a report of an injury to a patient in association with the presence of a hemostatic vascular clip in the MR environment.

Intravascular Coils, Filters, and Stents

Five of fifteen intravascular devices tested proved to be ferromagnetic.

■ Although they have shown deflection in the magnetic field, these devices usually become imbedded in the vessel wall after several weeks and are unlikely to become dislodged.

■ Therefore it is considered to be safe to perform MR imaging on most patients with intravascular devices, provided a reasonable period after implantation has elapsed.

Carotid Artery Vascular Clips

Each of five carotid artery vascular clamps displayed deflection in the magnetic field.

■ The deflection was mild when compared with pulsatile vascular motion within the carotid arteries.

■ Only the Poppen-Blaylock carotid artery clamp is contraindicated for MRI because of its large attractive response to the magnetic field.

Vascular Access Ports

Vascular access ports and catheters are bioimplants that are commonly used to provide long-term vascular administration of chemotherapeutic agents, antibiotics, analgesics, and other medications.

- Vascular access ports are implanted typically in a sub-cutaneous pocket over the upper chest wall with the catheters inserted in the jugular, subclavian, or cephalic veins. Smaller vascular access ports, which are less obtrusive and tend to be tolerated better, have also been designed for implantation in the arms of children or adults, with vascular access via an antecubital vein.

- Vascular access ports have a variety of inherent features (e.g., a reservoir, central septum, catheter) and are constructed from various types of materials including stainless steel, titanium, silicone, and various forms of plastic. Because of the widespread use of vascular access ports and associated catheters and the high probability that patients with these devices may require MR procedures, it was important to determine the MRI-compatibility of these bioimplants.

- Only three of the implanted vascular access ports tested had measurable deflection in the magnetic field. These deflections were thought to be insignificant to the applications of these ports. Therefore it is probably safe to image patients with implanted vascular access ports.

Artifacts from Implanted Vascular Access Ports

Even the *MRI-compatible* or *MRI-ports* made entirely from non-metallic materials are, in fact, observed on the MR images because they contain silicone. The septum portion of each of the vascular access ports typically is made from silicone. Using MRI, the Larmor precessional frequency of fat is similar to that of silicone (i.e., 100 Hz below fat at 1.5 T).

- Therefore silicone used in the construction of vascular access ports may be observed on MR images with varying degrees of signal intensity depending on the pulse sequence selected for imaging. Manufacturers of non-metallic vascular access ports have not addressed this finding during the advertising and marketing of their products.

- Vascular access ports made from nonmetallic materials are claimed to be MRI-compatible and invisible on MR images. However, if a radiologist did not realize that this type of vascular access port was present in a patient, the MR signal produced by the silicone component of the device could be considered an abnormality, or at the least, present a confusing image. This confusion may present a diagnostic problem for a patient being evaluated for a rupture of a silicone breast implant, because silicone from the vascular access port may be misread as an "extracapsular silicone implant rupture."

Heart Valves

Many heart valve prostheses have been evaluated for the presence of attraction to static magnetic fields of MR systems at field strengths of as high as 2.35 T. The majority of these prostheses displayed measurable yet relatively minor attraction to the static magnetic field of the MR system used for testing.

- Because the actual attractive forces exerted on these heart valves were minimal compared with the force exerted by the beating heart (i.e., approximately 7.2 N), an MR procedure is not considered to be hazardous for a patient who has any of the heart valve prostheses that have been tested. This includes the Starr-Edwards Model Pre-6000 heart valve prosthesis, which was previously suggested to be a potential hazard for a patient undergoing an MR procedure.
- With respect to clinical MR procedures, there has never been a report of a patient incident or injury related to the presence of a heart valve prosthesis.

Dental Devices and Materials

Many of the dental implants, devices, materials, and objects evaluated for ferromagnetic qualities exhibited measurable deflection forces, but only the ones that have magnetically activated components (i.e., held in place by magnets in the dentures and imbedded within the gums) present a potential problem for patients during MR procedures.

- The other dental implants, devices, and materials are held in place without magnetic components (such as pastes) generally do not cause problems for patients.

■ Although most devices are not significantly affected by the magnetic field, susceptibility artifacts can adversely affect image quality in MR, especially in gradient echo imaging.

Penile Implants

Only one of nine penile implants tested showed measurable deflection to the magnetic field. Two of these implants (the Duraphase and Omniphase models) demonstrated substantial ferromagnetic qualities when exposed to a 1.5 T static magnetic field of an MR system.

■ It is unlikely that a penile implant would severely injure a patient undergoing an MR procedure because of the relative strength of the magnetic field interactions associated with a 1.5 T MR system. This is especially the case considering the manner in which this type of device is used.

■ Nevertheless, it would undoubtedly be uncomfortable for the patient to undergo an examination using an MR system. For this reason, subjecting a patient with one of these particular penile implants to an MR procedure is inadvisable.

Otologic Implants

Three out of three cochlear implants were attracted to the magnetic field, are magnetically or electronically activated, and are contraindicated for MR imaging. Many patients with otologic implants have been issued a card that warns them to avoid MR imaging.

Ocular Implants

Of 12 ocular implants tested, four were deflected by a 1.5 T static magnetic field. The Fatio eyelid spring, the retinal tack made from martensitic (i.e., ferromagnetic) stainless steel (Western European), the Troutman magnetic ocular implant, and the Unitek round wire eyelid spring were attracted by a 1.5 T static magnetic field. A patient with a Fatio eyelid spring or round wire eyelid spring may experience discomfort but would probably not be injured as a result of exposure to the magnetic fields of an MR system. Patients have undergone MR procedures with eyelid wires after having a protective plastic covering placed around the globe along with a firmly applied eye patch. The retinal tack made from martensitic stainless steel and Troutman magnetic ocular implant may injure a patient undergoing an MR procedure, although no such case has ever been reported.

Intraocular Ferrous Foreign Bodies

Another concern of metallic implants in and around the eye is the potential problems resulting from intraocular ferrous foreign bodies. It is not uncommon for patients who have worked with sheet metal or who had been employed as a welder to have metal fragments or slivers located in and around the eye.

- Since the magnetic field exerts a force on ferromagnetic objects, a metal fragment in the eye could move or be displaced, which could cause injury to the eye or surrounding tissue.

- It is true that small intraocular fragments could be missed on a standard radiograph. However, a recent study demonstrated that metal fragments as small as $0.1 \times 0.1 \times 0.1$ mm were detected on standard radiographs.

- In addition, metal fragments from $0.1 \times 0.1 \times 0.1$ mm to $0.3 \times 0.1 \times 0.1$ mm were examined in the eyes of laboratory animals in a 2.0 T magnet. Only the $0.3 \times 0.1 \times 0.1$ mm fragments moved (i.e., rotated) but did not cause any discernable clinical damage.

- Although computed tomography (CT) is more accurate in detecting the presence of small foreign bodies, plain film radiography may be adequate in screening for intraocular ferrous foreign bodies of sufficient size to cause ocular damage.

Metallic Foreign Objects

When any possibly metallic foreign body is suspected to be in position within a patient, several factors must be reviewed before permitting the patient to undergo an MR examination. The presence of the metallic object or device within that patient must be confirmed, which is generally accomplished by the usage of radiographic studies, predominantly plain films.

- The location of the metallic object must then be determined to ascertain whether there are any anatomically sensitive structures (e.g., brain, lungs, major neurovascular bundles) in its vicinity. Even the risk of heating the

object is a concern, especially if the object is sufficient-
ly superficial (i.e., close) to the transmitting RF coil.

■ The mass of the object should be estimated to determine
whether it poses a potential threat to the patient in an
MR environment, since the potential forces exerted on
such a metallic object are determined in part by the
mass of the suspected ferromagnetic object.

■ Even the orientation of the object relative to the magnetic lines of force and its shape help to determine the
degree of possible risk for exposing the patient to an MR
system. For example, a weakly ferromagnetic object, with
its long axis parallel to the lines of force (as opposed to
perpendicular to them), such as certain inferior vena
caval filters, may pose less of a safety hazard than one in
which the lines of force lie vertically or perpendicular to
the long axis of the metallic device, implant, or object.

Bullets, Pellets, and Shrapnel

In some cases, a ballistics report can be obtained from local
authorities to determine the metallic content and trace metals
contained within ammunition. Although the majority of
ammunition has proved to be made of nonferrous materials,
ammunition made in foreign countries or produced by the mil-
itary has shown traces of ferromagnetic alloys. In an effort to
reduce lead poisoning in ducks, the United States government
has required the use of steel shot instead of lead, which could
produce a potential hazard in patients who have been shot
inadvertently.

■ It is advised to take extreme caution when imaging
patients with bullets or shrapnel and to be aware of the
location of these metals within the body.

Orthopedic Implants, Materials, and Devices

Each of 15 orthopedic implants tested showed no deflection
within the main magnetic field. However, magnetic and RF
fields can induce sufficient currents that can heat a large
metallic implant such as a hip prosthesis. It appears that this
heating is relatively low.

■ A majority of orthopedic implants have been imaged
with MR without incident.

Surgical Clips and Pins

Abdominal surgical clips are generally safe for MR imaging because they become anchored by fibrous tissue. Metallic implants also produce imaging artifacts in proportion to their size and can distort the image. Although it may not be necessary, it is a common practice to wait several weeks after surgery (i.e., 2 to 6 weeks, depending on whom you ask) before permitting postsurgical patients with surgical or vascular hemostatic clips to undergo MRI examinations. The rationale is that there may be mild ferromagnetic properties to these clips which, if only recently implanted, may not yet be firmly enough scarred in place to ensure that they would not be dislodged by their interactions with the static magnetic field of the MR imaging system. After several weeks, however, sufficient scarring is presumed to be present to permit a greater degree of assurance that the clips would not be substantially affected or moved by their interactions with the static magnetic field of the MR imager.

- Each surgical (or postsurgical case) should be evaluated on a case-by-case basis to ensure that the benefit of the MR procedure clearly outweighs any risk.

Halo Vests and Other Similar Externally Applied Devices

When planning to image a patient wearing a halo vest, several risk factors must be considered, including deflection and subsequent dislodging the halo, heating as a result of RF absorption, electrical current induction within the halo rings, electrical arcing, and severe artifactual consequences that could render the imaging acquisition useless.

- There are commercially available, nonferrous and non-conductive halo vests that are MR compatible. Therefore in light of the potential risks and hazards associated with halo vests, it may be advisable to identify the halo vest before proceeding with MR procedures.
- Although the halo itself may be made of nonferrous material such as titanium, in some cases the bolts that hold the halo frame together can be ferrous. For this reason, careful testing of the entire assembly with a hand-held magnet of considerable field strength (approximately 50 gauss), including the attaching bolts, should be completed before imaging the patient within the halo.

Electrically, Magnetically, or Mechanically Activated or Electrically Conductive Implanted Devices

Certain implanted devices are contraindicated for MRI because they are magnetically, electrically, or mechanically activated. These implants include cochlear implants, tissue expanders, ocular prosthesis, dental implants, neurostimulators, bone growth stimulators, implantable cardiac defibrillators, implantable drug infusion pumps, and the more commonly known cardiac pacemakers. (Pacemakers will be discussed later in more detail.)

- The functionality of these implants will be impaired by the magnetic field within the imager thus patients with these implants should not be imaged with MR.
- Devices that depend on magnetization to affix to the patient, such as magnetic sphincters, magnetic stoma plugs, and magnetic prosthetic devices, could be demagnetized and should be removed before (or should contraindicate) MRI.

Pacemakers

Cardiac pacemakers are an absolute contraindication for MRI. Field strengths even as low as 10 gauss may be sufficient to cause deflection or programming changes or to close the reed switch and convert a pacemaker to an asynchronous mode. Additionally, even patients in which the pacemaker has been removed, remaining pacer wires could act as an antenna and, by induced currents, cause cardiac fibrillation.

- Warning signs should be posted at the 5-gauss line to prevent the exposure of anyone with a pacemaker or other electronic implants.
- Pacemakers present potential problems to MR scanning from two points: motion of the pacemaker in strong static magnetic fields (e.g., 1.0 T), and modification of the function of the pacemaker, both temporarily or permanently, by the static magnetic field of the MR imager.
- Heating and voltages or currents can be induced in the pacemaker leads or in the myocardium during the MR imaging process. This is caused by the time-varying, RF magnetic fields of the imaging system during the MR imaging process, and can present potential problems.

It should still be considered contraindicated to scan any patient with a cardiac pacemaker in an MR scanner unless the following precautions are included:

- Integrated and coordinated approach with cardiology and knowledgeable personnel from radiology (and perhaps the Institutional Review Board or Human Rights Committee or both).
- Involvement and informed consent from the patient, which includes discussion of possible arrhythmias, pacemaker malfunction, and death
- Exceptionally strong indications that there is indeed a powerful clinical need for scanning this particular patient using MR technology.

In some cases, after the patient no longer needs the assistance of the cardiac pacemaker, it is removed. Although the pacer itself has been removed, in many cases the pacer wires are left in the patient. Canine studies indicate that during MR image acquisition in subjects whereby pacer wires are attached to the left ventricle, the heart can be paced in time with the TR (i.e., the time between RF pulses).

- In the past, imaging patients with residual pacer wires was contraindicated. Currently, many imaging facilities have found this effect to be negligible, thus they proceed with imaging patients with implanted wires if *and only if* the wires are cut short (i.e., flush with the skin) and there are no loops of wire outside the patient.
- Even with these requirements, such patients should be imaged with caution.

ASSESSING AND MONITORING

The Society for Magnetic Resonance Imaging adopted the following recommendation (Kanal E, Shellock FG, SMRI Safety Committee, 1992):

- "It is good practice for all patients undergoing magnetic resonance examinations to be visually and/or verbally monitored." This means simply that the technologist is to look at and talk to the patient before, during, and after the MRI procedure.
- If patients are unable to communicate with the technologist, then more than verbal and visual monitoring is sug-

gested. These patients may be sedated, comatose, unre-
sponsive, pediatric, hearing impaired, deaf, mute, have
weak voices, or they do not speak the same language.

■ All patients undergoing MR examinations who are
unable to communicate readily with the scan operator
and accompanying personnel should be physiologically
monitored by appropriate means.

The type of monitoring that is most appropriate is itself
dependent on the type of patient and examination being performed, as well as what type of equipment might be available
at the site. Such monitoring can include gross visual inspection
and monitoring of pulse rate, electrocardiogram (ECG), respiratory rate, pulse oximeter, capnometer, and temperature.

■ Numerous monitoring devices are presently available
that have been tested, have been found to be appropriate and safe for use in and around environments that
have high magnetic fields, and do not interfere with the
MRI process itself.

■ The specific type of monitoring that is to be performed
should be determined by the site. Suggestions include
pulse oxymetry (physiologic monitoring of respiration),
heart rate, blood pressure, or ECG, as clinically indicated. Furthermore, there are many clinical MR examinations that are being performed under sedation or even
general anesthesia, and the applications are growing in
number.

■ Appropriate patient monitoring during MR examinations
should be performed on all sedated or anesthetized
patients to control possible adverse reactions to the
drugs being used.

■ All clinical MR sites should have the appropriate monitoring equipment available before beginning an MR
examination of a patient who might require monitoring.

Studies that need to record ECG data for the purpose of gating also require the proper acquisition of the appropriate physiologic signal for accurate and timely representation of the desired
MR images. The use of MR-safe ECG electrodes is strongly recommended to ensure patient safety and proper recording of the
ECG in the MR environment. Accordingly, ECG electrodes have
been specially developed for use during MR procedures that pro-

tect the patient from these potentially hazardous conditions and that produce minimal MRI-related artifacts.

Sedated Patients in MRI

Sedated patients should be monitored by pulse oxymetry. The ECG leads that are used for cardiac gating are insufficient for monitoring such patients since the magnet-hemodynamic effect causes an elevation in the T-wave thus producing an artifact on the monitor. Furthermore, many sedation medications are respiratory depressants and it is therefore important to measure the oxygen saturation.

Claustrophobia

Although claustrophobia, as with other psychologic effects, appears less than critical compared with of other biologic effects of MRI, it is a condition that warrants mention. Radiofrequency (RF) heating, gradient noise, and the confines of the imager itself add to the possibility of claustrophobic reactions.

Although the majority of these effects are transient,

- There are several reported cases of patients who were not known to be claustrophobic before the MR examination but who had great difficulty in completing the examination and subsequently developed persistent claustrophobia. These patients required long-term psychiatric treatment.
- It is important to have controllable air movement within the bore of the magnet to maintain a comfort zone for patients. This factor, along with good patient contact and education, could help reduce claustrophobic reactions, which clearly is a safety concern in MRI.

CONTRAST AGENTS FOR MRI

To date, there are a number of contrast agents for MRI that have been approved by the FDA. These agents include paramagnetic (T1) agents (such as gadolinium and manganese) and superparamagnetic (T2) agents (such as iron oxide). Each of these agents has its own safety profile, but in general, both are relatively safe for patients. Of these aforementioned contrast agents, gadolinium is more widely used.

Gadolinium Side Effects and Reactions

Although the side effects of gadolinium chelates are minimal when compared with iodinated contrast agents, gadolinium has reportedly caused anaphylaxis and death in less than 1% of the patients injected.

- Gadolinium side effects usually include a slight transitory increase in bilirubin and blood iron, mild transitory headaches, nausea, vomiting, urticaria or rash, and in rare incidences, anaphylaxis and death.
- Between 1988 and 1993, approximately 5,000,000 intravenous injections of gadolinium have been administered, and only 17 cases of adverse events causing death had been reported.
- In general, anaphylactoid reactions are among the worst of the adverse events that a patient might experience and anticipate using these agents (with an incidence of approximately 1:100,000 to 1:500,000).
- Response times (from the onset of symptomatology to the arrival on scene with appropriate medical personnel) have been approximately 60 to 90 seconds.

Dose for Gadolinium

- All three gadolinium chelates (gadoteridol, gadopentetate dimeglumine, and gadodiamide) are administered by intravenous (IV) injection. Each injection of gadolinium is recommended to be followed by an injection with 5 cc saline flush. Gadolinium chelates (gadopentetate dimeglumine) restricts the injection rate to below 10 ml per minute. Intraarticular injection of gadolinium contrast agents is not found on any package insert.
- The effective dose of Gd-DTPA is 0.1 millimole per kilogram of body weight (mmole/kg), approximately 0.2 cc/kg or 0.1 cc/lb, not to exceed 20 cc. However, the FDA has approved one gadolinium chelate (gadoteridol) for triple-dose injection volumes. This dose, recommended on the package insert, allows for 0.1 mmole/kg followed by 0.2 mmole/kg up to 30 minutes after the first dose. This dosage is used to evaluate for single or multiple metastatic lesions in the brain.

Precautions for Gadolinium

Package inserts from Magnevist, Omniscan, and Prohance list no contraindications for the use of gadolinium chelates. However, there is a rather extensive list of precautions that should be reviewed by each person who administers the drug. These precautions include sickle cell disease, hemolytic anomalies, renal failure, allergies, and asthma, as well as pregnant and lactating mothers.

■ The side effects of gadolinium chelates are minimal; however, patient history should always be reviewed before the administration of this or any drug. Sickled red cells have been shown in studies to align perpendicular to the magnetic field. Some gadolinium chelates may possibly potentiate sickle cell alignment. Any patient with severely impaired renal function may require dialysis following contrast enhancement with gadolinium.

■ Pregnancy studies performed on rats and rabbits have indicated increases in spontaneous abortion (at 20 times the recommended dose), an increased incidence of post implantation loss (at 33 times the recommended dose), and an increase in spontaneous locomotor activity in offspring after 6 to 10 mmole/kg/day for 13 days (which is 20 to 33 times the recommended triple dose of 0.3 mmole/kg). Recent studies in pregnant baboons have revealed that the gadolinium can cross the placenta thus entering the amniotic fluid.

■ The fear is that the gadolinium can reside in the amniotic fluid and be swallowed by the fetus and subsequently secreted in the urine. The relative fear is that the gadolinium can come away from the chelate and become toxic to the fetus during the gestational period during which it is in direct contact with the developing fetus.

Iron Oxide Contrast Agents

There are contraindications for the use of iron oxide particles (Feridex) that include patients who cannot have iron. There are also side effects associated with this agent, including groin and back pain. Furthermore, imaging should be delayed at least 20 minutes after injecting this agent. (For more information about this agent, please refer to the package insert.)

Life-Threatening Situations

There have been numerous patients (at least two dozen to date) who have been placed in MRI systems (either intentionally or inadvertently) who have experienced life-threatening situations. There appears to be documentation that at least five of these have died.

- It should be stressed that in several of these cases, the cause of death is not known.
- Life-threatening situations include patients with contraindicated implants (intracranial aneurysm clip and cardiac pacemakers), contraindicated materials entering the scan room (projectiles), and lethal contrast or drug reactions.

Safety Precautions for Placement of Electrical Conductors

RF coils can be responsible for significant burn hazards caused by electrical currents produced in conductive loops. Faraday's law of induction states that when a magnet moves past conductive loops, voltages are induced within these loops. Equipment used in MRI such as ECG leads and surface coils should be used with extreme caution.

- Whenever surface coils or ECG leads are used, it is critical to avoid creating conductive loops within the imager to avoid antenna effects. Coils of wire and the patient have been known to create these loops.
- Cables that are not insulated can ignite tissue or clothing.
- Coupling a transmitting coil to a receiver coil may also cause severe thermal injury. For this reason, it is important that coil cables are not looped in the imager or do not touch the skin of the patient in two places. In the latter case, the patient completes the loop and runs the risk of obtaining significant burns.
- Routine checks of surface coils by the site's engineer should be performed to ensure proper function. It was

recommended by the New York Academy of Science at a conference during which they presented "Biological Effects and Safety Aspects of NMR," stating that wires used in MRI systems should be electrically and thermally insulated.

ENVIRONMENTAL CONSIDERATIONS: TEMPERATURE AND HUMIDITY

It is recommended that most imaging facilities be maintained at an ambient temperature of approximately 65° to 70° F and humidity of approximately 50% to 60%.

- The moderate temperature recommendation ensures proper functionality of the many computers that control the MR imagers.
- The intermediate humidity recommendation also ensures accurate operation of the computer system.
- An environment that is too hot will shut down the computer system, too damp will produce moisture, and too dry will produce static.
- Other temperature considerations exist with the magnet itself.
- Superconducting magnets are maintained at a temperature of 4° K, which is approximately –375° F.
- Permanent magnets should be maintained at a temperature between 68° and 72° F. These temperatures are imperative to maintain the magnetic fields in these imaging systems.

GAUSS LINE AND MAGNETIC FIELD STRENGTH

A secondary concern regarding the effects of the main magnetic field is the hazards inherent in siting of MR imagers.

- The static magnetic field has no respect for the confines of conventional walls, floors, or ceilings.
- The stray magnetic field outside the bore of the magnet is known as the fringe field.

Although most MR imagers today are shielded from the magnetic field so as to confine the fringe field to an acceptable location either within the scan room or, in the case of a mobile

MR system, to within the confines of the truck itself, the fringe field should be considered when the final siting decision is made. Even the field strength felt near the ceiling or on the floor below the imager must be considered when siting to prevent the untimely demise of a painter with a pacemaker who inadvertently climbed a ladder to paint the ceiling.

- The general public is generally restricted to the 5-gauss line. For this reason, most imaging systems are shielded to within 5 gauss within the wall surrounding the imager. For persons entering beyond this point, restrict all pacemakers and defibrillators, all magnetically activated implanted devices, or implanted devices that are themselves either magnetic or strongly ferromagnetic.

- If there is a history of metallic or possibly metallic structures that may have struck or entered the eye, then they are also restricted from the higher magnetic field strengths (even when they say that all metal was subsequently removed).

Magnetic Field Shielding

Fringe fields, however, can be compensated for by the use of magnetic field shielding. MR imagers can be shielded by either of two processes: passive shielding or active shielding.

- Lining the walls of the MR scan room with steel or concrete can accomplish passive shielding. This technique is low in cost and offers effective confinement of the magnetic field.

- Active shielding, a more expensive alternative, uses additional solenoid magnets outside of the cryogen bath providing smaller magnetic fields, which force the magnetic field lines of the main field to an acceptable location. Some imager manufacturers offer active shield magnets with stray fields in an area as small as one quarter of a tennis court. This facilitates siting of these systems such that space requirements are significantly less than unshielded systems.

RF Shielding

The RF used in clinical imaging is on the order of approximately 64 megahertz, which is similar to the frequencies used to broadcast ultrahigh frequency (UHF) and very high frequency (VHF) signals. To keep RF from leaving the MR scan room and to keep outside RF from entering, RF shielding known as a Faraday Cage can be used. Generally, this is accomplished by lining the MR scan room with cooper.

- For RF leaks leaving the room, the transmitted RF power from the MR scanner-transmitter coils apparently drops off approximately a thousand-fold at the bore of the MR scanner, as well as at an operator's console in the adjacent room.

- Therefore it is unlikely that any RF oscillating magnetic fields being transmitted during the MRI process could even be detected at the lengthy distance at which the typical operator console sits from the RF transmitter coils.

EMERGENCY PROCEDURES

In the event of a medical or technical emergency, it is recommended that the patient be removed from the MR scan room immediately.

- In the case of a medical emergency, the code team will need to administer to the patient, and since most of the crash cart items are magnetic, this procedure could become devastating if attempted in the presence of the strong magnetic field.

- In the case of a technical or equipment emergency, such as a quench or in the rare case of a fire, the patient should be removed to avoid any deleterious effects. In any case, the patient should be removed immediately from the MR scan room to avoid exacerbating the emergency.

QUENCH

To create an electromagnet, current is passed through the loops of a wire to create the magnetic field or to bring the field up to strength. To negate the effect of resistance in the wire, the wires are supercooled with substances known as cryogens, usually liquid helium. Helium cryogen keeps the magnet at a superconducting temperature, however, some systems use two cryogens: liquid helium and liquid nitrogen. In this case, the nitrogen merely keeps the helium cool. Helium may have problems associated with potential "boil off," but nitrogen is *deadly!*

■ Liquid helium is approximately −375° F or 4° K. To achieve this low temperature, helium gas is compressed. Approximately 750 liters of helium gas is used to make one liter of liquid helium, and most imaging systems use approximately 1000 liquid liters to fill the system.

■ Since helium gas is unstable, it is placed in an insulated vacuum such that these cryogens do not return to their gaseous state or "boil off." If these cryogens escape or come in contact with the environment, then "boil off" results.

■ This "boiling off" is known as a quench. During this quench, approximately 75 (liters of gas per liquid liter) × 1000 (total liters of liquid in the system) = 75,000 liters of helium gas can "boil off" into the scan room.

■ Remember that a quench that inadvertently vents into the magnet room will likely produce a "cloud" of condensing water vapor, which can be easily confused with smoke when viewed rapidly or from a distance. Many fire departments have rules and regulations of not being permitted into a smoke-filled environment without an oxygen tank strapped to the back of the firefighter. Therefore it is important to educate them in the anticipated appearances of a quench that may have at least partially vented into the magnet room so that they may proceed with appropriate caution and skepticism in such circumstances when arriving at the MR site (should they be called).

More importantly, the helium that enters the scan room will replace the oxygen that exists in the room, causing asphyxia or hypoxia. In addition, the "steam" that is formed from the boiling helium is rather cold thus frostbite or hypothermia can ensue.

■ It is strongly recommended that the patient be removed from the scan room immediately in the event of a quench.

■ Nitrogen can cause *death* if inhaled. For this reason, a properly ventilated room is a *must* in systems that use two cryogens.

EVACUATION

It is recommended that one should *never* attempt to "run a code" within the magnet itself. If *anyone* should, for any reason, attempt to place any ferromagnetic object, device, monitor, defibrillator, or similar object in the "heat of the emergency" on the patient, for example, within the active shield of the system, substantial trauma to the patient or health care personnel may inadvertently result.

- Identify an area for each MR imager, away from the static magnetic field of the imager, to which the patient would be evacuated so as to control and run a full code, if necessary. This action will help anyone involved to focus on providing emergent care to the patient without concern for the objects being brought into the area by other well-meaning but poorly prepared personnel who might respond to the emergency.
- It is better to handle an emergency in a carefully prepared manner, rather than to inadvertently create another emergency in the process.

BIOLOGIC CONSIDERATIONS

Although there are virtually no long-term, adverse biologic effects of extended exposure to MRI as a whole, separate components of the MRI process, including magnetic, gradient, and RF fields, should be examined for inconsequential and biologic effects, as well as following government recommendations.

RADIO FREQUENCY FIELDS

Exposure of the patient to RF occurs during MR examinations, as the hydrogen nuclei being imaged are subjected to an oscillating magnetic field. The source of this radiation is the RF coils that surround the patient inside the magnet bore.

Specific Absorption Rate
MR imaging systems cannot measure RF exposure. Therefore it is necessary to measure RF absorption, which is manifested as tissue heating. The health-related criterion of RF heating is the patient's ability to dissipate excess heat. Energy dissipation

can be described in terms of specific absorption rate (SAR). SAR is expressed in watts per kilogram (W/kg), a quantity that depends on induced electric field, pulse duty cycle, tissue density, conductivity, and the object radius.

- Knowing the patient's weight and the pulse sequence parameters allows for proper monitoring of SAR. Care must be taken in recording the patient's actual weight to ensure that the SAR does not exceed the permitted levels.
- SAR can be used to calculate an expected increase in body temperature. In an average examination, the body temperature can be expected to rise from approximately $0°$ to $2°$ C.

FDA Guidelines for RF Exposure

- The FDA sets guidelines for MR imaging. In the United States, the recommended SAR level for imaging is 4.0 W/kg (whole body), 3.2 W/kg (head), and 8 W/kg (small volume).
- In Canada, the recommended SAR level is 2.0 W/kg. Recently, the FDA has reclassified MRI facilities. Sites that are studying the safety of scanning at SAR values above 4.0 W/kg whole-body average are no longer required to limit their capabilities for proton imaging. Sites using research software such as spectroscopy may still require approval.
- For noninvestigational MRI sites, new modifications have been established to allow more slices per scan on body imaging. The FDA has acknowledged MRI as an established diagnostic tool with recognized risks that are well controlled by the design and use of the equipment.

Studies have shown that patient exposure up to three times the recommended levels produced no serious adverse effects, despite the elevations of skin and body temperatures. As body temperature increases, we also expect to see an increase in blood pressure and heart rate. One study performed showed no significant increase in these vital signs. Although these effects appear insignificant, patients having compromised thermoregulatory systems may not be candidates for MRI. In addition, the areas of the body with the inability to dissipate heat, such as the eyes and the testicles, have been evaluated independently and in standard pulse sequences, have shown no significant increase in temperature. Corneal temperatures were shown to increase from 0° to 1.8° C. However, as faster imaging sequences arise, these areas may need to be re-evaluated.

Potential Bioeffects to RF Irradiation

Because the energy level of frequencies used in clinical MR imaging is relatively low when compared with x-rays, visible light, and microwaves, the predominant biologic effect of RF irradiation absorption is the potential heating of tissue. Although nonthermal effects have been reported, to date these effects have not been confirmed. As an excitation pulse is applied, some nuclei absorb the RF energy and enter the high-energy state. As nuclei relax, they give off this absorbed energy to the lattice. In frequencies below 100 MHz, 90% of absorbed energy results from tissue currents (eddy currents in tissues) induced by the magnetic component of the RF field.

- As the frequency is increased, absorbed energy is increased, thus heating of tissue is largely frequency-dependent. For this reason, in MR systems operating below 1.0 T, RF heating becomes less of a concern.

There are four ways that humans control temperature (thermoregulation): convection, conduction, radiation, and evaporation. All four of these methods depend on the availability of surface area to move heat from the center (core) of the patient outward so as to be released into the environment and away from the organism.

- In general, it certainly holds true that the greater the available surface area (actually, the surface-area-to-volume ratio), the greater the ability of the patient to handle a power or heat load and to dissipate it more rapidly to the surrounding lattice or background environment.

- RF effects increase with an increase in RF pulses; thus new rapid fast spin echo (FSE) sequences are of greater concern for this effect.

STATIC FIELD STRENGTH

The main magnetic field is also known as the static magnetic field. This field is responsible for the alignment of nuclei for MRI. In solenoidal electromagnets, the field is generally horizontal, whereas in permanent magnets, the field is generally vertical.

Projectiles

Ferromagnetic metal objects can become airborne and act as rockets known as projectiles in the presence of the strong static magnetic field. Small ferromagnetic objects such as paper clips and hairpins will have a terminal velocity of over 60 mph when pulled into a 1.5 T magnet. Even surgical tools such as hemostats, scissors, and clamps, although made of a material known as *surgical stainless steel*, are highly attracted to the main magnetic field.

- Oxygen tanks are also highly magnetic and are attracted to the static magnetic field. They should never be brought into the scan room. However, there are nonferrous O_2 tanks that are MR-compatible.

- Sandbags have also become suspect since some are filled not with sand, but with "steel shot," which is highly magnetic. It is recommended that all objects be tested with a handheld bar magnet for attractive potential before entering the MR scan room.

- It is also advised that all nursing, housekeeping, fire department, emergency, and MRI personnel be educated to the potential risks and hazards of the static magnetic field.

- Signs should be posted to deter possible entry into the scan room with ferromagnetic objects.

- Metal detectors are available, but can, in some cases, offer a false sense of security. For this reason, most imaging facilities keep the general public well behind the 30-gauss line.

Prescreening for Projectiles

The "missile effect" refers to the capability of the fringe field component of the static magnetic field to attract ferromagnetic objects (e.g., oxygen tanks, tools) that may be subsequently drawn into the MR system by considerable force.

- The "missile effect" can pose a significant risk to the patient inside the MR system or anyone who is in the path of the ferromagnetic object that is attracted by the magnetic fringe field.
- In extreme cases, the high field, superconducting magnet may need to be "quenched" for MR systems with superconducting magnets or turned-off to extract sizable ferromagnetic objects from the MR systems, resulting in substantial financial loss from down time, replacement of cryogens, and so on.
- Therefore every MRI site should establish a protocol for detecting metallic objects before allowing individuals to enter into the MRI environment to avoid injuries or other problems related to missile effects.

To guard against these potential catastrophes, the immediate area around the MRI system should be clearly demarcated, labeled with appropriate warning signs, and secured by trained staff members who are cognizant of MR-related safety procedures. In addition, patients and other individuals who must enter the MR environment should be carefully screened for objects that may be involved in the "missile effect."

Tesla

The strength of the magnetic field, expressed by the notation (B) or, in the case of more than one field, the primary field (B_0) and the secondary (B_1), can be measured in one of three units: gauss (G), kilogauss (kG), and tesla (T). Gauss is a measure of low magnetic field strengths. For example, the strength of the earth's magnetic field is approximately 0.6 G. T, conversely, is the unit used to measure higher magnetic field strengths. The three units of measure can be compared using the following equation:

$$1\ T = 10\ kG = 10{,}000\ G$$

Static Fields Below 2 T

- Although no biologic effects have been observed in human subjects at field strengths below 2 T, reversible abnormalities have been noted on ECGs. An increase in the amplitude of the T-wave is noted on the ECG from the *Magnetic Hydrodynamic Effect or the Magnetic Hemodynamic Effect.* This effect is produced when a conductive fluid (in this case, blood) moves across a magnetic field. This effect is also proportional to the strength of the magnetic field and tends to present problems for cardiac gating techniques in high-field scanners. Gating problems occur when the system recognizes and tries to "trigger" from the T-wave rather than the R-wave. Image quality suffers as a result of insufficient cardiac gating. However, no serious cardiovascular effects have been observed in patients.

Another concern is the potential heating of patients exposed to static fields. Two studies were performed independently during which patients were exposed to field strengths of 1.5 T for 60 minutes and 20 minutes, revealing minimal increases in body temperatures of 0.10° and 0.03° C, respectively.

Static Fields Above 2 T

- Some reversible biologic effects were observed on human subjects exposed to 2 T and above. These effects included fatigue, headache, hypotension, and accounts of irritability. Another concern of magnetic field strengths above 2 T include effects from magnetic interaction energy and cell orientation. Certain molecules such as DNA and cellular sub-units such as sickled red cells have magnetic properties that vary with direction. This effect is biologically important at a field strength of 2 T because of the twisting force or torque that is exerted on these molecules. Even at 1.5 T, most imaging facilities try to delay imaging patients in sickle cell crisis, at least until after the crisis to avoid potential aligning of sickled red cells with the magnetic field.

Biologic Effects

The primary concern with the static (main) magnetic field is the possibility of potential biologic effects. In nature, the magnetic field associated with the earth does have significant effect on lower life forms. The orientation of magnetostatic bacteria and the migratory patterns of birds are influenced by the 0.6 G magnetic field that surrounds the earth.

■ During MRI, small electrical potentials have been observed in large blood vessels that flow perpendicular to the static magnetic field. However, even at 10 T, no adverse effects have been noted on the ECGs of squirrel monkeys.

■ The majority of studies show no effects on cell growth and morphology at field strengths below 2 T. Data accumulated by the National Institute for Occupational Safety, the World Health Organization, and the State Department regarding employees exposed to high levels of microwave radiation at the United States Embassy in Moscow, revealed no evidence of leukemia or other carcinogenesis. However, the *New England Journal of Medicine* (1982) reported an increase in leukemia in men exposed to electric and magnetic fields in the state of Washington from 1950 to 1979. Although similar effects were noted in New York in 1987, no evidence of adverse effects have been noted in persons working with linear accelerators who are exposed to static magnetic fields. These reports of potential carcinogenesis seem controversial since many of the study's procedures have been criticized.

FDA GUIDELINES FOR STATIC MAGNETIC FIELDS

Because many studies appear to mark a difference between results of field strengths below 2.0 T and above 2.0 T, the FDA recommendations were such that clinical imaging could be performed in magnetic field strengths up to 2.0 T. Recently, the FDA has amended the recommendation to 4.0 T for clinical imaging. Today, clinical imaging of patients can thus be performed in imagers of field strengths of up to and including 4.0 T.

GRADIENT MAGNETIC FIELDS (TIME-VARYING MAGNETIC FIELDS)

All MRI systems are equipped with a set of resistive wire windings known as gradient coils. Gradients provide position-dependent variation in magnetic field strength and are pulsed on and off during and between RF excitation pulses.

■ The purpose of these gradients is to spatially encode information contained in the emitted RF signal. However, in doing so, they create a time-varying magnetic field (TVMF).

Biologic Effects of TVMF

There have been a large number of studies performed on the biologic effects from TVMF since they exist near power transformers and high-voltage lines in today's environment.

■ The health consequences are not related to the strength of the gradient field, but rather, to changes in the magnetic field that causes induced currents.

■ During MRI, the safety concern involves the nerves, blood vessels, and muscles that act as conductors in the body. According to Faraday's law of induction, changing magnetic fields will induce electric currents in any conducting medium. Induced currents are proportional to the material's conductivity, the rate of change of the magnetic field, and the radius of the inductive loop.

■ During MRI, this effect is determined by factors such as pulse duration, wave shape, the repetition pattern, and the distribution of the current in the body. The induced current is greater in peripheral tissues since the amplitude of the gradient is higher away from isocenter.

Biologic effects vary with current amplitude from reversible alterations in vision to irreversible effects of cardiac fibrillation, alterations on the biochemistry of cells, and in some cases, inspired fracture union. Studies also indicate stimulation of bone healing by inducing an electric field and then altering the magnetic field to the direction of the desired area of interest.

■ Effects experienced in MRI range from mild cutaneous sensations, to involuntary muscle contractions, to cardiac arrhythmias.

■ Visual effects occur when retinal phosphenes are stimulated by induction from TVMF. Light flashes or "stars in one's eyes" are the end result. These studies were performed on human and animal subjects and were performed at field strengths up to 3.0 T.

Acoustic Noise

The switching of gradients during the imaging sequence causes activation and deactivation of coils. Therefore the activation and deactivation of TVMF in the presence of a static magnetic field results in torque or rotational forces on the gradient coils. These forces are believed to result primarily in vibration and secondarily auditory noise that is audible during the MR imaging process.

■ This noise is audible only during the time that the gradients are being used (i.e., during image acquisition). As we activate and deactivate the current through the gradient coils during image acquisition, we create a significant amount of acoustic noise. Although noise levels on most commercial imagers are considered to be within recommended safety guidelines, it can cause some reversible and irreversible effects.

■ These effects include communication interference, patient annoyance, transient hearing loss, and in patients who are susceptible to hearing impairment, permanent hearing loss. Acceptable and inexpensive means for the prevention of hearing loss is the regular use of disposable earplugs. A more expensive alternative would be *antinoise* or destructive noise apparatus, which not only reduces noise, but also permits better communication between the operator and the patient.

FDA Recommendations for TVMF

The FDA has chosen to follow the auditory safety guidelines adopted by the Occupational Safety and Health Administration (OSHA), which varies the permitted decibel level based on the time duration of exposure.

■ For example, 102 decibels would be the maximum permitted for a 1-hour, continuous noise exposure. It is well documented that one of the factors that determines hearing loss is the duration of exposure to the noise.

■ It is important to remember that absolute magnitude of the noise, although important, should be viewed only in combination with duration of exposure to determine potential harmful results to patients who are exposed.

■ A sequence that uses steeper and rapidly altering gradients (e.g., the echo planar technique) may produce a greater amplitude than another sequence, but may also result in substantially decreased exposure times. Both of these techniques should be evaluated together when determining patient safety.

■ For time varying effects, the FDA limit for exposure was, at one time, limited to a gradient strength of 6.0 T per second. Since this has proven to cause little or no long-term adverse effects, the FDA has recently changed this limit to one in which the patient experiences discomfort. Time-varying effects increase with an increase in gradient speed. Therefore new rapid gradient sequences such as echo planar imaging (EPI) sequences are of greater concern for this effect.

Future Safety Considerations

Several types of investigational bioimplants, materials, devices, and objects are presently undergoing clinical trials. These experimental items incorporate electrically, magnetically, or mechanically activated mechanisms that could pose a hazard to patients referred for MR procedures.

■ A magnetically controlled heart valve has been described that can be activated so as to stay open or closed, depending on the requirements of the circulatory system. This prosthetic heart valve uses a small electromagnet that surrounds a ferromagnetic disk within the valve mechanism. Movement of the valve is regulated by the field generated, by the electromagnet, and the resulting force on the disk. Obviously, the operation of this magnetically controlled heart valve would be seriously compromised if a patient with this implant were exposed to the electromagnetic fields of an MRI system.

■ An endovascular catheter used for aneurysm embolization has been described that uses an external magnetic field for guidance of the device. Because this device must be retained in the aneurysm and because inadvertent movement by the magnetic fields of an MR system is possible, the presence of this device would likely be contraindicated for a patient referred for an MRI procedure.

Another experimental technique used for embolization of blood vessels has been described such that ferrous particles are introduced into the vascular system and guided by an external magnetic field to the site of the abnormality. When this technique of embolization is used in the clinical setting, patients who have undergone this procedure must be identified because of potential risks associated with the displacement of the ferrous particles during exposure to the magnetic fields of MRI systems.

The clinical applications of magnetic microspheres used for the targeted and controlled release of medications or diagnostic agents to single or multiple organs are being evaluated presently. These magnetic microspheres typically are injected into the arterial system near the targeted organ and then subjected to an externally applied magnetic field gradient ranging from 0.55 to 0.80 T to position them in or near the tissue. The magnetic fields associated with MR systems would likely disrupt the placement of the magnetic microspheres. Furthermore, the magnetic microspheres may become dislodged from the intended organ. Obviously, MRI procedures should not be performed on patients with magnetic microspheres until the safety implications have been determined.

The remote magnetic manipulation of a small ferromagnetic "seed" used for delivery of drugs, focal hyperthermia, or other treatments to brain tissues has been described. This ferromagnetic "seed" is maneuvered to a precise location within the brain using static magnetic fields at field strengths less than those used for clinical MR procedures.

■ Displacement of the ferromagnetic seed is likely to occur when a patient with one of these bioimplants is subjected to the magnetic fields associated with an MR system.

As previously mentioned, there are various MRI systems that are being used on an ongoing investigational basis with static magnetic field strengths of 3.0 and 4.0 T. Notably, an 8.0 T MRI system is now in operation at Ohio State University. Few of the biomedical implants or devices have been evaluated for safety in association with these MRI systems. Therefore an extremely cautionary approach is required whenever individuals with ferromagnetic objects are examined using these particular MRI systems with high field strengths.

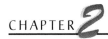

Introduction to Clinical MRI Procedures

Chapter at a glance

INTRODUCTION TO CLINICAL MRI

Before the introduction and use of magnetic resonance imaging (MRI), there were several methods used to evaluate the human body for anatomy and pathologic conditions. Methods such as plain film radiography were used to evaluate bone, computed tomography (CT) to evaluate brain and intra-abdominal organs, ultrasound to evaluate retroperitoneum and the pelvis, pneumoencephalography to evaluate ventricular anatomy, angiography to evaluate the vascular system, and exploratory surgery to evaluate anything that could not be seen by these methods. All of these techniques were invasive procedures. Some used ionizing radiation or the introduction of iodinated contrast agents and some invaded the body surgically. Because of its high soft tissue contrast, multiplanar capability, and noninvasive technique, MRI has in many cases become the imaging modality of choice for evaluating the body.

In the previous sections, the physics principles that prove the possibility of MRI were discussed. Although these principles may appear somewhat abstract, and although comprehension of these principles appears to be nonessential for everyday imaging, they hold the keys that open the doors to clinical MRI. In this section, the physics principles will be presented as reality in clinical imaging protocol examples and image acquisition strategies. The intention is to assist the MRI technologist in maximizing image quality and minimizing artifacts without sacrificing overall imaging time. Understanding the basic physics and using that knowledge to increase diagnostic specificity of the image can help to reach this goal. This section describes an introduction to clinical MRI.

PATIENT PREPARATION FOR CLINICAL MRI

There are several steps that should be performed before the actual imaging acquisition in MRI. The first step is to ensure proper patient screening techniques for both clinical history and metal implants so as to avoid hazards and artifacts and to guarantee the acquisition of optimal imaging sequences. The next step is to provide optimal radio frequency (RF) coil selection and proper patient positioning to ensure quality MR imaging. (*For general patient screening tips, see the safety section. For specific clinical tips, see each clinical section.*)

Special Considerations for Pediatric Patients

As with other imaging modalities, MR imaging of children poses obstacles not often encountered when imaging adults. Since children are easily frightened, and the appearance of most MR systems can be intimidating, care should be taken to provide a secure atmosphere for a successful imaging examination.

- A calm and confident manner generally transfers tranquility to the child.
- When this fails to work, sedation and immobilization techniques can be used for children up to the age of 10 years.
- MR systems make loud sounds during image acquisition that can be startling to adult patients and terrifying to children. Therefore earplugs or headphones should always be used for pediatric patients.
- The first imaging challenge in pediatric imaging is simply to complete the examination before the child moves, or for sleeping children, before they wake up.
- The second challenge is to complete the appropriate examination by evaluating small human bodies that are not completely formed. For example, in children under the age of 1 year, the brain is not yet myelinated.
- For this reason, special imaging sequences of the brain are selected to optimize the visualization of brain tissue, such as longer time to the echo (TE) for T2-weighted (decay time) images or inversion recovery (IR) with intermediate (500 ms) time between the inverting pulse and the excitation pulse (TI) for T1-weighted (recovery time) images.

Choosing the Right Protocol

Pulse sequence parameters (appropriate to properly evaluate the body and possible lesions) and imaging options (to enable virtually artifact-free images of the human body) are selected on the basis of anatomy and suggested pathologic condition.

- As in other diagnostic imaging modalities, one view (i.e., one set of images) is insufficient to evaluate patients in

MRI adequately. For this reason, a series of imaging acquisitions, known as a *protocol*, is selected for each patient to be studied with MRI.

■ Typically, T1-weighted images are used primarily to evaluate anatomy since they provide high signal-to-noise and T2-weighted images are used to evaluate pathologic conditions as a result of their high intrinsic contrast. Therefore, to evaluate the body thoroughly for lesions, both T1- and T2-weighted images are usually acquired.

PARAMETERS FOR IMAGE CONTRAST IN MRI

When we image at specific times during the relaxation processes (T1 = recovery time and T2 = decay time), we can acquire images with different levels of contrast (i.e., some structures appear bright and others appear dark).

■ For MR imaging, there are parameters that we cannot change, such as the T1 recovery time, the T2 decay time, and the proton density (PD). These parameters are known as intrinsic parameters (the parameters we cannot change).

■ Therefore to make images that look quite different in MR, we change the parameters that we can change, such as the time between RF pulses or the repetition time (TR), the time between the RF pulse and the time we sample the signal or the time to the echo (TE), and other parameters (TI and flip angle). These parameters are known as extrinsic parameters (the parameters we can change).

■ During MRI, we manipulate the extrinsic parameters to make images that exploit the intrinsic features. These images are known as T1-weighted images, T2-weighted images, and PD-weighted images.

To exploit contrast differences, we control the extrinsic parameters. These parameters can be used whereby TR goes with T1 and TE goes with T2. For example, decreasing TR provides more T1 information, and increasing TE provides images with more T2 information. Images that have been acquired with parameters chosen to exploit T1 are known as T1-weighted images, whereas images acquired for T2 are known as T2-weighted images.

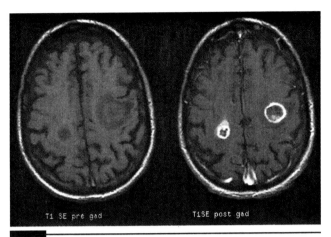

Figure 2-1 This example demonstrates T1 SE images acquired before *(left)* and after *(right)* contrast enhancement. In this case, the metastatic lesions enhance with gadolinium since the gadolinium causes the breakdown in the BBB that occurs around the lesions.

T1 Image Contrast

On T1-weighted images, the T1 contrast follows the order of T1 relaxation differences. On these images, tissues with short T1 times are bright indicating fat and tissues with long T1 times are dark indicating water (Figure 2-1).

- T1-weighted images use TR to manipulate the amount of T1 recovery that occurs between successive RF pulses.
- T1-weighted images use a short TR. A short TR (approximately 500 ms) is chosen such that T1 recovery (remember, that T1 times range from about 150 ms for fat and 2000 ms for water at 1.5 T) is in progress. In this case, a TR of 500 ms is in the middle of the T1 recovery times.

T2 Image Contrast

On T2-weighted images, contrast follows the inverse order of T2 decay differences. On these images, tissues with long T2 (water) appear bright and tissues with short T2 (fat) appears dark (Figure 2-2, *left*).

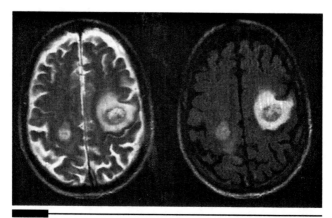

Figure 2-2 This example demonstrates a T2 FSE acquisition *(left)* and a FLAIR *(right)*. Note the metastatic lesions in the brain and compare the unenhanced and enhanced images (see Figure 2-1).

- T2-weighted images use TE to manipulate the amount of T2 decay that is allowed between excitation and the signal echo.
- A long TE (approximately 100 ms) is chosen such that T2 decay is in progress (remember, T2 times range from about 50 ms in fat and 200 ms in water at 1.5 T). In this case, a TE of 100 ms is in the middle of the T2 decay times.

Proton Density Image Contrast

On PD-weighted images, contrast follows the order of PD. On these images, tissues with high PD (water and fat) appear bright.

- PD-weighted images use TE to manipulate the amount of T2 decay that is allowed between excitation and the signal echo and TE to determine the amount of T1.
- A short TE (approximately 20 ms) is chosen such that T2 decay has not begun (remember, T2 times range from 50 ms in fat and 200 ms in water at 1.5 T). A long TR (over 2000 ms) is chosen whereby T1 decay is done. (Remember, T1 times range from approximately 150 ms in fact and 2000 ms in water.) In this case the T1 is virtually done and the T2 has not begun, thus contrast is governed by the number of mobile water protons.

Pulse Sequences

To acquire images with various image contrasts, we use various types of pulse sequences. Remember that a pulse sequence is a series of RF and gradient pulses that occur in a given order based on the parameters we choose. There are a number of pulse sequences available on imaging systems today. These pulse sequences include spin echo, fast spin echo, inversion recovery, and gradient echo. *(For more information about the physics of pulse sequences, refer to the section on pulse sequences.)*

Spin Echo Sequences

The majority of spin echo (SE) sequences use a 90° RF pulse followed by a 180° refocusing pulse. (Remember, any two RF pulses can create a spin echo; however, the 90°/180° combination is most efficient.) In these sequences, the 180° pulse refocuses the signal while correcting for inhomogeneities, chemical shift, and susceptibility. In this sequence, one line of k-space (the number of phase encoding steps = # PEs) is filled in each TR period. Scan time = TR × # PEs × NSA. The number of signals averaged (NSA) is the number of times each PE line is filled.

- To acquire an SE image whereby T1 contrast prevails, a short TR (approximately 500 ms) and a short TE (approximately 20 ms or less) can be selected. With these parameter choices, T1 is in progress (short TR) and T2 has not essentially begun (short TE). These images are generally used for anatomic information. On T1-weighted images, tissues with short T1 times (fat and gadolinium enhancement) appear bright. Because gadolinium shortens the T1 time within a lesion, T1-enhanced images can also be used to visualize abnormalities.

- To acquire an SE image whereby PD contrast prevails, a long TR (over 2000 ms) and a short TE (under 20 ms) can be chosen. With these parameter choices, T2 has essentially not begun (short TE) and T1 is nearly complete (long TR). On PD-weighted SE images, tissues with high PDs (almost everything) appear bright. These images are generally used for anatomic and pathologic information. *(For a PD image, see the spine and musculoskeletal sections.)*

■ To acquire an SE image whereby T2 contrast prevails, a long TR (over 2000 ms) and a long TE (over 100 ms) can be chosen. With these parameter choices, T2 is in progress (long TE) and T1 is nearly complete (long TR). On T2-weighted images, tissues with long T2 times (water and many lesions) appear bright. These images are generally used for pathologic information.

Fast Spin Echo Sequences

Fast spin echo (FSE) sequences use a 90° RF pulse followed by multiple 180° refocusing pulses. In these sequences, the 180° pulses refocus signal while correcting for inhomogeneities, chemical shift, and susceptibility. In this sequence, multiple lines of k-space (# PEs) fill in each TR period. The number of lines is known as the echo train length (ETL). Scan time = (TR × # PEs × NSA) ÷ ETL (see Figure 2-2).

■ A T1-weighted FSE sequence has a short TR and short effective TE. When acquired for T1 information, FSE sequences should be acquired with a short ETL. This will minimize the blurring that can occur on FSE sequences.

■ A PD-weighted FSE sequence has a long TR and short effective TE. When acquired for PD information, FSE sequences should be acquired with a short ETL. This will minimize the blurring that can occur on FSE sequences.

■ A T2-weighted FSE sequence has a long TR and long effective TE. When acquired for T2 information, FSE sequences should be acquired with a long ETL. On FSE images with a long effective TE, blurring is generally not an issue.

Inversion Recovery Sequences

Inversion recovery (IR) sequences use a 180° inverting pulse followed by a 90° RF excitation pulse followed by one single or multiple 180° refocusing pulses. When IR sequences are acquired with single refocusing pulse, it is a variation of the SE sequence; with multiple lines, it is a variation of the FSE sequence. Today, most IR sequences are acquired as a variation of a FSE sequence and are generally acquired for T1 or PD information. The time between the inverting pulse and the excitation pulse is known as the TI. TI is chosen for the image contrast desired.

■ Short TI inversion recovery (STIR) technique uses an inversion time to correspond to the time it takes fat to regrow to the null point. For STIR images, the TI time corresponds with the T1 time of fat for a given field strength. Therefore, for a STIR sequence acquired in a 1.5 T magnet, the TI time should be approximately 150 ms. In this case, fat can be suppressed on images with T1 information. Therefore STIR can be used to suppress the signal from fat. *Caution:* STIR can also suppress the signal form gadolinium-enhancing lesions. *(For a STIR image, see the musculoskeletal section.)*

■ Another type of inversion recovery sequence is FLAIR (fluid attenuated inversion recovery. FLAIR sequences are acquired with long TR and short TE and a long TI time. TI times vary with field strength but can be approximately 2000 ms at 1.5 T. The inversion time matches the time for fluid to regrow to the null point. For FLAIR images, the TI time corresponds with the T1 time of water for a given field strength. For a FLAIR sequence acquired in a 1.5 T magnet, the TI time should be approximately 2000 ms. In this case, water can be suppressed on images with PD information. Therefore FLAIR can be used to suppress the signal from water (Figure 2-3).

Gradient Echo Sequences

Gradient echo (GE) sequences use a variable RF pulse followed by a gradient pulse. In these sequences, the gradient pulse refocuses signal but does not correct for inhomogeneities, chemical shift, and susceptibility. GE sequences are notorious for susceptibility artifacts, but since flip angle is manipulated, TRs can be shorter thus scan times can be shorter. In this sequence, one line of k-space (the number of phase encoding steps = # PEs) is filled in each TR period. Scan time = TR × # PEs × NSA (see Figure 2-3) (Figure 2-4, *right*).

■ For fast T1 information, GE images with short TR (faster scan time), large flip (more T1 information), and short TE (less T2 Information) can be acquired. To clean up the steady state or T2* effect on the image, we randomize or spoil it away, which can be done with gradients or with additional RF pulses. This technique can provide rapid T1 images for acquisition during contrast enhancement. In addition, by manipulating the TE in these images, we can acquire images *in phase* or *out of phase* (see Figure 2-3).

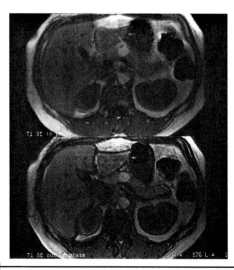

Figure 2-3 This example demonstrates T1 GE images acquired in phase *(upper)* and out of phase *(lower)*. Note the etching artifact surrounding structures that are fluid-filled surrounded by fat.

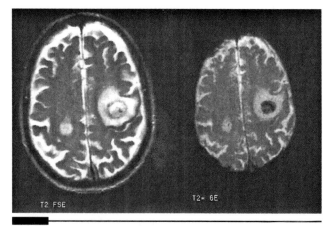

Figure 2-4 This example demonstrates a T2 FSE acquisition *(left)* and a T2* GE *(right)*. Note the metastatic lesions in the brain and compare the unenhanced and enhanced images (see Figure 2-1) and with the PD and T2 (see Figure 2-3). The low signal within the lesion noted on the GE image indicates the presence of blood products. On the GE image, the susceptibility artifact is a result of iron in the blood.

■ For T2* information, GE images with short TR (faster scan time), small flip (less T1 information), and long TE (more T2 Information) can be acquired. Also, during the acquisition of GE acquisitions, we use gradients and no 180° RF pulse. During the first little flip pulse, we tip the magnetization partially into the transverse plane. After that, some recovery occurs and we tip again. At this time, a little more is tipped and a little recovers. Eventually, we reach a condition whereby what we tip is what recovers. At this time, we have reached a condition known as *steady state*. At steady state we build up transverse magnetization, which provides T2 information. In addition, since we did no clean up of the "bad stuff" or inhomogeneities in the image, we gain an image known as T2* image (see Figure 2-4).

PARAMETERS FOR SIGNAL-TO-NOISE AND RESOLUTION

The relationship between the MR signal and the background noise is simply referred to as the signal-to-noise ratio (SNR). By evaluating the SNR, overall image quality can be assessed. It would be best to omit the noise completely, but this is not feasible. Therefore to increase the ratio between the signal and the noise, it is possible to use parameters, which are under user control, to increase the signal or decrease the noise thus increasing the ratio. The following chart can be used as a quick reference of these parameters.

Parameters	SNR
TR	Increase TR increases SNR
TE	Decrease TE increases SNR
Field strength	Increase static magnetic field (B_0) increases SNR
Signal averages	Increase NSA increases SNR
Bandwidth (BW)	Narrow BW increases SNR
Receiver coil	Smaller coils increases SNR
Voxel size	Increase voxel size increases SNR

High-Resolution Imaging

In some anatomic regions, *high-resolution imaging* techniques are required such that small structures are resolved, one from another. To achieve high spatial resolution, images are acquired with small voxels, achieved by selecting small field of view (FOV), thin slices, and a high imaging matrix (more phase or frequency encoding steps). Since high-resolution imaging requires the use of small voxels, there is a reduction in the SNR. In addition, since high-resolution imaging is usually low in signal, small voxel imaging techniques are not generally used in images that have low intrinsic SNR.

Voxel Size Determinants	
FOV	Increase FOV increases SNR and decreases resolution
Matrix	Increase matrix within the FOV decreases SNR and increases resolution
Slice thickness	Increase slice thickness increases SNR and decreases resolution

MR Scan Time

Modification of parameters that influence the quality of the signal may be costly because all imaging parameters are interrelated. These parameters are known as trade-off parameters. Some imaging parameters, while increasing signal, also increase imaging time, decrease resolution, or change image contrast. It is often up to the operator to select an optimal set of parameters suitable for each individual imaging challenge.

There are no faster or slower MR imagers. In all systems scan time is dependent on:

- TR
- Number of phase encodings (NPE)
- Number of NSAs
- Number of slices (NSL) in three-dimensional or single-slice image
- ETL in FSE of the number of shots in echo planar imaging (EPI)

When scan times take longer on one system when compared with another, one of these parameters has been increased. Occasionally, in an attempt to increase either SNR or spatial resolution or to alter image contrast, overall imaging time may increase. It is important to realize that patient cooperation is essential in optimal MR imaging. Therefore every effort is made in MRI to keep scan time to the minimum while keeping image quality high.

In two-dimensional imaging or single-slice acquisitions

$$\text{scan time} = TR \times N_{PE} \times NSA$$

In three-dimensional imaging

$$\text{scan time} = TR \times N_{PE} \times NSA \times N_{SL}$$

In FSE imaging

$$\text{scan time} = TR \times N_{PE} \times NSA \div ETL$$

In echo planar (EPI) imaging

$$\text{scan time} = TR \times NSA \times N_{shots}$$

Protocols are often selected on the basis of desired image contrast, optimal SNR, spatial resolution, and overall imaging time.

CREATING ARTIFACT-FREE IMAGES

It does not matter how conscientious the MR technologist is, unwanted artifacts almost always occur in MRI. Artifacts can occur as a result of the imaging process itself, such as sampling artifacts (e.g., truncation, aliasing), from RF interference (outside or within the scan room), or from motion. Fortunately, there are a number of imaging options (and tricks) that can be employed to compensate for these artifacts. These options, however, are not without cost, which can range from a slight decrease in the number of available slices per sequence to a significant increase in scan time. With each option, there is a trade-off cost. This section will briefly discuss common artifacts and imaging options to improve quality along with trade-off costs and penalties.

Physics Artifacts

Physics artifacts stem from such things as magnetic field inhomogeneities, usually caused by metal, and differences in frequency between proton spins, such as fat and water. Artifacts from inhomogeneities are called *susceptibility artifacts,* and artifacts from different frequencies are known as *chemical shift artifacts.*

Susceptibility Artifacts

When metals in the magnetic field cause inhomogeneities and create distortion artifacts in MR images, these artifacts are believed to be a result of the susceptibility effect.

- Susceptibility artifacts appear as an area of signal void usually surrounded by an area of hyper signal or anatomic distortion or both.
- The size of the artifact is dependent on the size and type of metal. Ferromagnetic metals create large disruptions in magnetic fields and subsequently, large artifacts.
- However, the same size particle of a nonferrous metal would create a smaller artifact.
- For images of metal artifacts, see Figure 1-1.

Occasionally, susceptibility artifacts are helpful for diagnosis. Older blood products such as hemosiderin contain iron and produce susceptibility artifacts.

- In these cases, blood within the lesion will appear black. GE pulse sequences acquired with long echo times can be used to enhance these effects.
- Also, large voxel imaging (i.e., images acquired with large FOV, small matrix, or thick slices) will increase intravoxel dephasing and increase susceptibility effects.
- For images of susceptibility artifact from blood, see Figure 2-4.

Chemical Shift Artifacts

Nuclei bound in different sites within an atom demonstrate different resonant frequencies in a magnetic field. This effect is known as *chemical shift*. For example, the hydrogen bound to oxygen in water has a slightly different frequency than hydrogen bound to carbon in fat.

- Frequency differences (i.e., chemical shift) are less at lower field strengths. Since frequency differences are less at lower and mid-field strengths, chemical shift artifact is negligible in images acquired in lower field strengths.
- Since frequencies vary slightly in these tissues, MR signals can be *mismapped* on images, acquired at high field strength, in areas where fatty and fluid-filled structures are side-by-side inside the body and are in the same voxel. This type of mismapping appears as a high signal-intensity area and a low signal-intensity area beside the water-filled structure surrounded by fat.
- Chemical shift artifact increases as gradient amplitude decreases. Gradient amplitude decreases with decreased FOV or with wider BW.

Chemical shift artifact can be used to help delineate structures in the abdomen.

- This technique is known as out-of-phase imaging.
- This technique was discussed in the T1 GE section earlier in this chapter.
- To evaluate an image with chemical shift artifact, see Figure 2-3.

Motion Artifacts

Since the MR sampling process can be long relative to the physiologic motion, motion artifacts are a common problem on MR images. Artifacts of this type occur as streaking across the phase encoding direction and are known as *phase ghosting*.

- Phase ghosting artifacts can be a result of movement such as peristalsis, respiration, pulsatile blood flow, and patient motion.
- Artifact causing motion can be either *periodic* (repetitive motion over time) or *aperiodic* (random motion).
- *Fast scanning* techniques help to minimize the artifactual effects of peristalsis, as well as respiratory motion, especially when used in association with breath-holding techniques.
- Other imaging options to minimize the effects of physiologic motion include cardiac or respiratory triggering or gating, gradient moment nulling, saturation pulses, fat-suppression techniques, and multiple SNAs.
- To evaluate motion artifact, refer to the prostate image in the pelvis section.

TYPES OF FDA-APPROVED CONTRAST AGENTS

Contrast agents in MRI have evolved from nothing to a plethora of agents, which include agents that are familiar to most MRI technologists, as well as agents that are still under investigation.

- Gadolinium is most widely used and is a paramagnetic agent.
- Gadolinium is also considered to be a T1 enhancement agent, since gadolinium shortens T1 times of tissues (bright on T1 images).
- Gadolinium also shortens T2 (dark on T2 images).
- For an enhanced image, see Figure 2-1.

Mechanism of Action

Gadolinium has the effect on tissue by influencing the local magnetic field and changing the relaxation times of the tissues in the vicinity. In these cases, gadolinium has the effect of shortening T1 and T2 relaxation times.

Effects on the Image

Since gadolinium shortens T1 and T2, there is a change in image contrast noted on the image.

- On T1-weighted images, whereby tissues with short T1 times, appear bright. Tissues with shortened T1 times appear bright.
- On T2-weighted images, whereby tissues with long T2 times, appear bright. Tissues with shortened T2 times appear dark.
- *For more detailed information about gadolinium and its particular effect in the body, see each clinical area.*

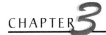

CHAPTER 3

Imaging Procedures: Head and Neck Imaging

Chapter at a glance

INTRODUCTION TO HEAD AND NECK MRI

Before the early 1970s, methods used to evaluate the brain abnormalities included invasive procedures such as pneumoencephalography to evaluate ventricular anatomy and angiography to evaluate the vascular system. In the 1970s, an imaging technique called computed tomography (CT) took the imaging world by storm by providing transaxial images of brain tissue, optimized when acquired after the injection of iodinated contrast agents. Although magnetic resonance imaging (MRI) was also in its infancy in the mid 1970s, image quality was poor and acquisition time for MRI was long relative to CT. As techniques for MRI improved and imaging times became more suitable for clinical imaging, MRI has, in many cases, become the modality of choice to visualize brain anatomy and most brain abnormalities.

Standard Protocols for Imaging of the Brain

Pulse sequence parameters (appropriate to evaluate brain tissue and possible lesions properly) and imaging options (to enable virtually artifact-free images of the brain) are selected on the basis of anatomy and suggested pathologic conditions of the brain. As with other diagnostic imaging modalities, one view or set of images is insufficient to evaluate patients in MRI adequately. Generally, T1- and T2-weighted images are acquired in several imaging planes for optimal imaging of the brain. For this reason, a series of imaging acquisitions, known as a *protocol*, is selected for each patient to be studied with MRI.

Imaging Planes for Brain Imaging

For brain imaging, the selected imaging planes (or views) are chosen for proper display of the anatomy and suggested abnormalities within the brain.

- Because the anatomy of the brain is displayed adequately in sagittal plane, sagittal T1-weighted, short TR (repetition time) and TE (time to the echo), localizer images are acquired to establish landmarks.
- Most imaging facilities follow the T1 sagittal *localizer* with a series of T2- and PD-weighted or FLAIR (fluid attenuated inversion recovery) images in the axial plane.
- Frequently, postgadolinium sequences are acquired in the axial and coronal planes. Incidentally, coronal images can also be acquired for temporal lobes (for seizures), pituitary, and internal auditory canal (IAC) imaging.

Image Contrast for Brain Imaging

Typically, T1-weighted images are used primarily to evaluate anatomy since they provide high signal-to-noise, and T2-weighted images are used to evaluate pathologic conditions because of their high intrinsic contrast. For this reason, a series of imaging acquisitions, known as a *protocol*, is selected for each patient to be studied with MRI.

- Therefore to evaluate the brain thoroughly, T1-weighted images (generally without and with contrast), PD (FLAIR), and T2-weighted images are usually acquired.
- T1 information is generally acquired with spin echo (SE) pulse sequences for brain imaging. Pulse sequence choices are generally selected by the capabilities of the imaging system, image quality, and scan time desired.
- T2 and PD information can be acquired in a number of ways such as SE, fast spin echo (FSE), gradient echo (GE), or echo planar (EPI). (For cases in which FSE or FLAIR sequences are unavailable on a particular imaging system, conventional SE sequences can be substituted for T2 and PD images of the brain, however, with longer imaging times.) Today, most facilities study the brain with T1 SE localizer in the sagittal plane, T2 FSE in the axial, and FLAIR in the axial plane.
- For the evaluation of lesions, either intraaxial (inside the blood brain barrier [BBB]) or extraaxial (outside the BBB), gadolinium contrast agents can be administered and images can be acquired in one or more imaging planes (sagittal, axial, or coronal, depending on the location of the lesion).

Additional Brain Sequences for Hemorrhage, Stroke, or Vascularity

Additional imaging sequences can be used to evaluate vascular lesions both inside and outside the head. Generally these sequences are variations of GE sequences.

- For hemorrhage, a T2* GE can be acquired with large voxel size and longer TE to increase susceptibility effects.
- For the evaluation of vascular lesions, either three-dimensional time of flight (TOF) or three-dimensional phase contrast (PC) MR angiography can be acquired.
- For the evaluation of stroke (infarct), fast GE sequences (e.g., EPI) can be acquired for diffusion or during dynamic contrast enhancement for perfusion.
- For the evaluation of brain function—**blood oxygenation level dependency**—images can be acquired. These are known as functional MRI (FMRI).

ANATOMY AND PHYSIOLOGY OF THE BRAIN

There are a number of anatomic structures that are important for the technologist to understand so as to evaluate lesions in the head accurately. The brain is composed primarily of gray and white matter. The significance to the technologist is that some lesions reside in the white matter, such as multiple sclerosis (MS) plaques, and some on the gray-white interface, such as metastatic lesions. In general, the white matter is the inside of the brain and the gray matter makes up the periphery or cortex (Figures 3-1 through 3-4).

- White matter is composed primarily of myelin. White matter tracts allow for electrical messages to travel through the brain.

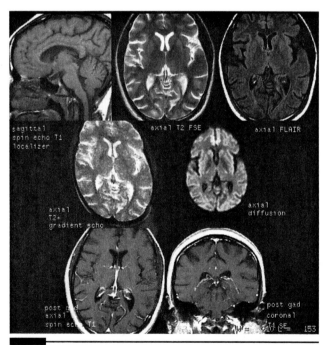

Figure 3-1   Brain protocol. This series represents a typical brain imaging sequence. In this series, the sagittal localizer *(upper left)*, axial T2 *(upper middle)*, FLAIR *(upper right)*, gradient echo *(middle left)*, diffusion *(middle right)*, postgadolinium axial T1 *(lower left)*, and postgadolinium coronal *(lower right)* are demonstrated.

■ The gray matter or cortex is responsible for functionality of the body, such as motor skills, and sensory functions, including vision, smell, sight, and hearing. There are several gray matter structures within the brain. These gray matter structures are known as the basil ganglia.

■ Also within the brain is a ventricular system through which cerebrospinal fluid (CSF) is produced and stored.

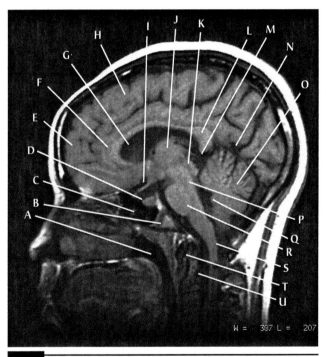

Figure 3-2 Brain anatomy demonstrated in the sagittal plane. Note the anatomic locations annotated on the sagittal image of the brain. *A,* nasopharynx; *B,* clivus; *C,* sphenoid sinus; *D,* pituitary gland; *E,* frontal lobe; *F,* corpus callosum (genu); *G,* anterior horn of the lateral ventricle; *H,* parietal lobe; *I,* optic chiasma; *J,* thalamus; *K,* cerebral aqueduct (aqueduct of Sylvius); *L,* corpus callosum (splenium); *M,* cisterna ambiens; *N,* tentorium cerebellum; *O,* cerebellum; *P,* medulla oblongata; *Q,* fourth ventricle; *R,* pons; *S,* spinal cord; *T,* anterior arch of C1; *U,* dens (odontoid of C2).

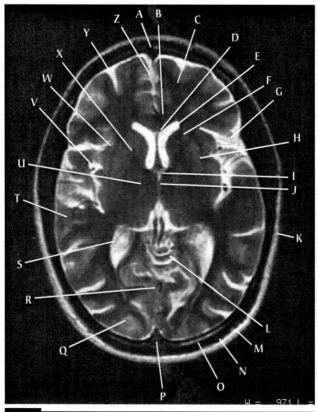

Figure 3-3 Brain anatomy demonstrated in the axial (transverse) plane. Note the anatomic locations annotated on the axial image of the brain. *A*, superior sagittal sinus; *B*, corpus callosum (genu); *C*, frontal lobe; *D*, septum pellucidum; *E*, anterior horn of the lateral ventricle; *F*, caudate nucleus (head); *G*, sylvian fissure; *H*, lentiform nucleus (putamen and globus pallidus); *I*, interventricular foramen; *J*, third ventricle; *K*, subcutaneous fat; *L*, vermis; *M*, cortical bone (skull outer table); *N*, fat in bone marrow; *O*, cortical bone (skull inner table); *P*, superior sagittal sinus; *Q*, occipital lobe; *R*, vessel; *S*, posterior horn of the lateral ventricle; *T*, parietal lobe; *U*, thalamus; *V*, claustrum; *W*, external capsule; *X*, internal capsule; *Y*, sulcus; *Z*, longitudinal fissure (inside is the falx cerebri).

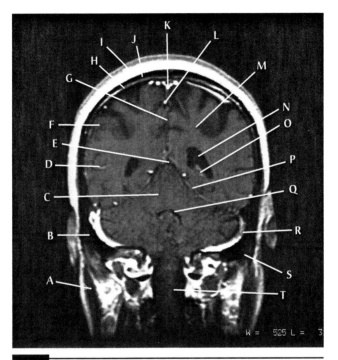

Figure 3-4 Brain anatomy in the coronal plane. Note the anatomic locations annotated on the coronal image of the brain. *A,* masseter muscle; *B,* mastoid air cells; *C,* cerebellum; *D,* sylvian fissure; *E,* cisterna ambiens; *F,* sulci; *G,* longitudinal fissure; *H,* fat in bone marrow (high signal); *I,* subcutaneous fat; *J,* cortical bone; *K,* superior sagittal sinus; *L,* falx cerebri, *M,* parietal lobe; *N,* body of the ventricle; *O,* choroid plexus; *P,* tentorium; *Q,* fourth ventricle; *R,* transverse sinus; *S,* mastoid air cells; *T,* spinal cord.

Patient Set-Up and Positioning for Brain Imaging

To image the brain, patients are positioned supine, and pads are placed under the knees to ensure patient comfort. Comfortable patients are generally less agitated and yield high-quality images. It is also recommended that all patients be given earplugs or headphones to minimize the effects of gradient noise.

Patient Screening for Brain Imaging
All patients should be screened to avoid contraindications for MRI.

- For brain imaging, patients who have altered mental status may pose a problem for conventional questionnaires and patient interviews.
- Furthermore, patients who have had previous aneurysms should be considered as a potential contraindication for MRI with ferrous intracranial vascular clips.
- A thorough screening of family members or referring physicians may be required so as to avoid contraindications for MRI.

Coil Selection and Positioning for Brain Imaging
In most cases, for brain imaging, patients are positioned within a transmit-receive head coil.

- Most head coils have a quadrature configuration to allow for optimal signal-to-noise ratio (SNR).
- Patients are positioned supine with the head all the way up and centered within the head coil.
- Pads can be placed under and on both sides of the head for immobilization and comfort.

Landmarking for the Standard Brain Protocol
For standard brain imaging protocols, patients are positioned such that the head is centered to the center of the head coil. At this time, the landmark is established and the patient's landmark is sent to the isocenter of the magnet.

- The longitudinal (right to left) landmark is along the mid-sagittal plane of the patient (right down the middle of the patient and along the nose).

- The coronal (anterior to posterior) landmark is in the middle of the head at approximately the level of the external auditory meatus (EAM).
- The axial (superior to inferior) landmark is at the glabella (or at the level of the eyebrows).

Imaging Options for Brain Imaging

There are several artifacts that commonly appear on brain images. These artifacts include phase ghosting or motion (flowing blood, CSF, or patient motion), aliasing (wrap around or phase wrap), and chemical shift (around the globes of the eyes). These artifacts can be minimized by the following imaging options:

- To reduce flow motion artifacts, apply saturation pulsed inferior to the field of view (FOV) to aid in the reduction of artifacts caused by flow coming into the FOV.
- Gradient moment nulling (GMN) or flow compensation (FC) can be used on T2 acquisitions to aid in the reduction of flow motion artifacts caused by slower flow found within the FOV. However, GMN will produce bright vessels and in doing so may enhance phase ghosting around the vessels.
- Employ cardiac or peripheral gating if pulsatile vascular motion is still a problem, especially in the temporal lobes where these artifacts occur as a result of pulsatile blood flow in the circle of Willis and in the ventricles of the brain.
- Artifacts caused by patient motion can be reduced by using rapid imaging techniques or by sedating the patient.
- Aliasing can be reduced with oversampling techniques.
- Chemical shift artifact is generally not a problem unless imaging of the orbits is required.

INDICATIONS FOR CONTRAST AGENTS FOR BRAIN IMAGING

To gain both pathologic and anatomic information, an axial T1-weighted, short TR and TE series scanned through areas of interest can be acquired following an injection of contrast agents. At this time, gadolinium is the paramagnetic contrast of choice for brain imaging.

- Gadolinium contrast agents can be used to enhance lesions within the head, both inside (intraaxial) and outside (extraaxial) the BBB. Gadolinium will not cross an intact BBB, but will enhance lesions in which the BBB is compromised (or broken down).
- Gadolinium contrast will cause signal enhancement in extraaxial areas (outside the BBB). Extraaxial structures or structures that can normally enhance include the pituitary gland, pineal gland, infundibulum, falx cerebri, slow flowing vessels, choroid plexus, and the pineal gland.
- Its usefulness in the brain is in suggested infarction, infection, inflammation, and tumor, preoperative and postoperative, as well as before and after radiation therapy.

Standard Dose and Administration for Gadolinium

The United States Food and Drug Administration (FDA) has approved gadolinium chelate for use as a contrast agent in MRI. It is recommended that gadolinium chelate be administered intravenously over several minutes followed by a 5 cc saline flush.

- Standard dose for gadolinium is 0.1 mmole/kg of body weight.
- This translates to a dose of 0.2 cc/kg.
- This amount translates to a dose of approximately 0.1 cc/lb or 10 cc for a 100 pound patient.
- Some contrast agents (gadolinium) have been approved for higher dose for the evaluation of metastatic lesions in the brain. *In this case, the dosage would be a single dose followed by a double dose for a total equaling a triple dose.*

Mechanism of Action and Effects of Gadolinium on Brain Images

The effect of gadolinium is that it shortens the T1 and T2 times of tissues near the area that the contrast resides.

- In T1-weighted images, tissues with short T1 times appear bright. In general, lesions have a long T1 time since they are composed primarily of free water. Gadolinium shortens the T1 time of the lesions allowing them to appear bright on T1-weighted images. As the result, intraaxial lesions such as metastatic lesions, meningiomas, gliomas and infarcts will enhance because of their breakdown in the BBB.

- Perilesional edema will not enhance since BBB breakdown is limited to the periphery of the brain insult (tumor lesion or infarct). Edema is an excessive accumulation of fluid that leaks into normal brain tissue.

- Gadolinium also shortens the T2 time of tissues. As a result, T2 images acquired in the head after the introduction of gadolinium will demonstrate a reduction in signal or appear darker. To evaluate perfusion imaging in the brain T2*, EPI sequences are acquired before, during, and after contrast enhancement. The normal brain (that which gains perfusion) will get progressively darker, and an area of infarct (that which does not perfuse), will remain bright.

INDICATIONS FOR HIGH-RESOLUTION BRAIN IMAGING

When imaging smaller structures within the head, high-resolution techniques are required such that fine anatomic structures can be resolved from each other. These areas include the IACs, pituitary, cranial nerves, and the orbits, among others.

- For this reason, parameters such as smaller FOV, thinner slice thickness, or larger matrix are selected for imaging. The tradeoff for such selections is a decrease in SNR. High-resolution techniques may require an increase in the number of signal averages (NSA) or a narrow bandwidth (BW) to buy back the loss in signal. An increase in the NSA results in an increase in scan time. By increasing NSA, the SNR can be increased without compromising voxel size, however, the cost is longer imaging times.

- Coil selection may be limited to the head coil such that signals deep within the brain are detected. For this reason, usually a quadrature transmit-receive head coil is used.

Internal Auditory Canal

When evaluating a patient for tinnitus, hearing loss, or vertigo, the evaluation of the IACs is indicated.

- Specifically for IACs, high-resolution images acquired in the coronal and axial planes are optimal.
- Within the IACs are the seventh and eighth cranial nerves. These cranial nerves originate on the pons.

Pituitary

If a patient is to be evaluated for maturity or developmental abnormalities, this may be an indication for MRI of the pituitary gland.

- For the evaluation of the pituitary gland, high-resolution images in the coronal and sagittal planes are optimal.
- Connecting to the superior aspect of the pituitary gland to the hypothalamus is the pituitary stalk of infundibulum. Both the pituitary gland and the infundibulum enhance with gadolinium since they are normally outside the BBB.

Orbit

Evaluating a patient for visual disturbances may be an indication for MRI of the orbits.

- For the evaluation of the orbits, high-resolution images in the axial and sagittal oblique planes are optimal. Furthermore, for increased SNR, surface coils can be placed over the eyes.
- The optic nerve extends from the globe of the orbit to the optic chiasma. This optic nerve is the second cranial nerve.

Soft Tissue Neck

Because of its high soft tissue contrast, MRI is useful for the evaluation of lesions of the neck (Figure 3-5).

- For the evaluation of lesions in the soft tissue of the neck, patients are positioned supine with a coil placed over the anterior neck. Images are generally acquired in the sagittal and axial planes. Occasionally, coronal images are useful for the evaluation of lesions near the vessels of the neck.
- As with the head T1-, T2-, and contrast-enhanced sequences are generally acquired.

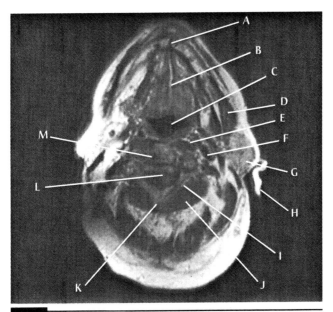

Figure 3-5 Neck anatomy demonstrated in the axial plane. Note the anatomic locations annotated on the axial image of the neck. (For further evaluation of neck anatomy, see the sagittal series in the cervical spine section.) *A,* mandible; *B,* tongue; *C,* trachea; *D,* masseter muscles; *E,* carotid artery; *F,* jugular vein; *G,* parotid gland; *H,* ear; *I,* lamina; *J,* erector spine muscles; *K,* spinous process; *L,* spinal cord; *M,* vertebral artery.

- There are many causes for motion artifacts on neck images, including swallowing, pulsatile flow motion, and respiration, since the anatomy of the neck includes (from posterior to anterior) the spine-esophagus-trachea (SET). To minimize motion artifacts in the neck caused by swallowing, patients should be instructed not to swallow during image acquisition. To reduce flow motion artifacts, saturation pulses can be applied inferior and superior to images.

CHAPTER 4

Spine Imaging Procedures

Chapter at a glance

INTRODUCTION TO SPINE MAGNETIC RESONANCE IMAGING

As late as the early 1980s, the best way to evaluate the spine for anatomy or abnormalities was with the use of myelography. Myelography is an invasive procedure that requires the injection of contrast agents into the subarachnoid space by way of a lumbar or lateral cervical puncture. Following these contrast injections were plain film radiographs or computed tomography (CT) of the spine. Potential risks of this procedure include reactions to contrast agents, infection from injections, and radiation from x-rays producing risks of long-term biologic effects for many patients.

Because of the high soft-tissue contrast and multiplanar capabilities, magnetic resonance images of the spine are, in most cases, superior to images acquired with myelography or even myelographic CT. Sagittal, axial, coronal, and oblique imaging planes help to display the anatomy of the spine on MR images. Multiple oblique views can be acquired through intervertebral disk spaces. Superior high soft-tissue contrast provided by magnetic resonance imaging (MRI) of the spine demonstrates structures such as bone marrow, spinal cord, cerebrospinal fluid (CSF) in the subarachnoid space, and nerves near the spinal cord. In this way, MRI provides phenomenal visualization of the anatomy of the spine and surrounding structures.

STANDARD PROTOCOLS FOR IMAGING THE SPINE

As with the head, pulse sequence parameters (appropriate to evaluate the spine and possible lesions properly) and imaging options (to produce virtually artifact-free images of the spine) are selected based on anatomy and suggested abnormalities of the spine. As with other diagnostic imaging modalities, one view (one set of images) is not sufficient to evaluate patients in MRI adequately. Typically, T1-weighted images are used primarily to evaluate anatomy since they provide a high signal-to-noise ratio (SNR), and T2-weighted images are used to evaluate pathologic conditions because of their high intrinsic contrast. Therefore to evaluate the spine thoroughly, both T1-weighted images (generally without and with contrast) and T2-weighted images are usually acquired. For this reason, a series of imaging acquisitions, known as a *protocol*, is selected for each patient to be studied with MRI.

Imaging Planes for Spine Imaging

For spine imaging, the selected imaging planes (views) are chosen to properly display the anatomy and suggested abnormalities within the spinal column, spinal cord, or spinal canal.

- Because the anatomy of the spine is displayed adequately in the sagittal plane, sagittal T1-weighted, short TR-TE (recovery time–time to the echo) *localizer* images are acquired to establish landmarks.

- A series of high-resolution T1, T2, and proton density (PD)–weighted fluid attenuated inversion recovery (FLAIR) images in the sagittal plane are useful to evaluate anatomy and abnormalities of the spinal structures.
- To provide an additional view, a series of T2 and FLAIR images in the axial (or axial oblique) plane are generally acquired.
- Coronal views are generally not acquired for spine imaging, especially in adults whereby normal kyphosis and lordosis will degrade acquisitions in the coronal plane.

Image Contrast for Spine Imaging

To evaluate the spine properly, high-resolution imaging is generally required. For this reason, pulse sequences that provide a high SNR are optimal. The capabilities of the imaging system, image quality, and the desired scan time generally determine which pulse sequence is to be used.

- Typically, T1-weighted, spin echo (SE), (short TR-TE) images are used primarily to evaluate anatomy since they provide a high SNR (that can be traded for high resolution) in acceptable imaging times. Generally, T1 is acquired with SE, however, if faster imaging is needed, it can be acquired with fast spin echo (FSE) or gradient echo (GE).
- T2 information can be acquired in a number of ways, such as SE, FSE, GE, or echo planar (EPI). For the spine, T2 information is generally acquired with FSE (long TR-TE) since this sequence offers high SNR in rapid imaging times long echo train length (ETL).
- PD information can be acquired with SE, FSE, GE, or FLAIR images. FSE may not be considered for PD information in the spine since blurring can occur on FSE images with short TE times. However, if FLAIR images are required, FSE acquisitions allow imaging to be completed in more acceptable imaging times.
- For high-resolution, axial T2 or T2* images, generally, a three-dimensional (3-D), GE sequence is employed. The 3-D acquisition allows for thinner slices and therefore higher resolution.

Additional Spine Sequences for High Resolution

Additional imaging of high-resolution, 3-D, GE sequences can be used to evaluate the spinal cord and the neural foramina through which the nerves traverse. For 3-D (volume) acquisitions, thin slices allow for high-resolution imaging. In addition, these sequences can be reformatted to evaluate the spinal cord and nerve roots in any imaging plane.

Anatomy and Physiology of the Spine

When imaging the spine with MRI, the anatomic structures that are visualized include not only the bony structures such as the vertebral bodies, but also cartilaginous structures, intervertebral disks, muscles, blood vessels, nerves, tendons, epidural and subarachnoid space, and the spinal cord (Figure 4-1). Numerous structures are important for the technologist to understand to evaluate structures in the spine accurately.

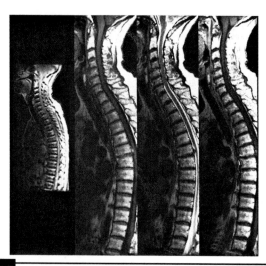

Figure 4-1 **Spine protocol.** This series represents a typical spine imaging sequence. In this series, the sagittal GE localizer (*left*), sagittal SE T1 (*second from left*), sagittal FSE T2 (*second from right*), and sagittal T1 SE postgadolinium (*right*) are demonstrated. Generally, axials are also acquired for spine imaging. These axial views can be found later in this chapter.

- On MR images, cortical bone is not observed. However, bone marrow within the vertebral body is visualized because of its high fat and water content. For this reason, vertebral bodies are visualized by MRI.
- Because soft-tissue structures are involved in a number of insults that occur within or around the spine, it is important to be familiar with the normal anatomy of the spine and the surrounding structures (Figure 4-2).

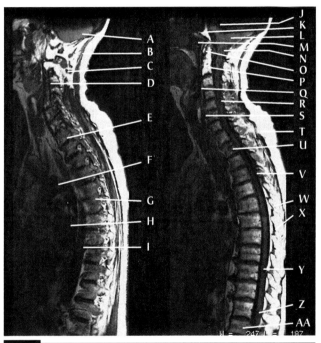

Figure 4-2 Spine anatomy demonstrated in the sagittal plane. Note the anatomic locations annotated on this mid-sagittal image of the complete spine. *A,* cerebellum; *B,* neck muscles; *C,* facet joint; *D,* vertebral artery; *E,* neural foramina; *F,* aortic arch; *G,* disk; *H,* left atrium; *I,* descending thoracic aorta; *J,* pons; *K,* clivus; *L,* cerebellar tonsils; *M,* nasopharynx; *N,* spinal cord; *O,* anterior arch of C1; *P,* dens (odontoid of C2); *Q,* epiglottis; *R,* posterior longitudinal ligament; *S,* anterior longitudinal ligament; *T,* spinatus tendon; *U,* T2; *V,* spinal cord; *W,* epidural fat; *X,* ligamentum flavum; *Y,* cerebrospinal fluid; *Z,* conus medullaris; *AA,* L1.

- The spinal cord is made up of gray and white matter, similar to the brain. However, dissimilar to the brain (gray on the outside and white on the inside), the spinal cord has white matter on the outside and gray matter on the inside.

- In this section, the cervical, thoracic, and lumbar spine will be discussed. When these sections are introduced, pertinent anatomy will be annotated.

Patient Set-Up and Positioning for Spine Imaging

Patients who have back pain may be more comfortable with *pads* under the knees. Patients with cervical spine abnormalities may need to have some form of padding under the neck. This factor poses a slight problem since coil coupling is important. The coil should be as close to the patient as possible for maximal signal detection. Therefore pads under the coil or a small roll under the natural lordotic areas of the spine may help to ensure patient comfort without sacrificing the SNR.

Patient Screening for Spine Imaging

As with all MR procedures, *patient screening* is important when imaging the spine. It is important to screen for ferromagnetic intraocular foreign bodies, aneurysm clips, and pacemakers. It is also important to be aware of previous surgeries and injuries within and around the spine.

- In particular, screening becomes critical when patients have had spine fusions or spinal wiring before the early 1970s. Occasionally, it has been demonstrated that fusion wires may be ferromagnetic and could be contraindicated for MR.

- In addition, shrapnel or bullets near the spinal cord that exhibit torque within the magnetic field can cause spinal cord injury.

Special Considerations for Patients with Spinal Cord Injuries

Patients imaged with MRI to rule out spinal cord compression may require special handling to avoid further spinal cord injury.

- Patients with cord lesion should be handled with caution since improper patient motion can lead to a complete spinal cord compression, which can cause further damage to the cord. For this reason, delicate patient handling of these patients should be considered.
- In many cases, MR examinations of the entire spine can be lengthy procedures, especially without the use of a phased-array or a multicoil-array apparatus. In these cases, *fast scanning* GE techniques can be considered to keep scan times down. As always, because GE techniques tend to be loud, *earplugs* should be provided for patients to minimize the possibility of acoustic damage.
- These patients can be in severe pain and may require *premedication*, which may require physiologic monitoring during the MR procedure. In addition, patients will yield better images when they are made comfortable enough to tolerate the examination.

Coil Selection and Positioning for Spine Imaging

For most cases in which spine imaging is required, patients are positioned supine and on a phased-array spine coil.

- Because the spinal cord can be approximately 40 cm long in the average adult, complete spine imaging poses a significant challenge.
- In early MR procedures, it was difficult to evaluate the entire spine since the field of view (FOV) was limited to *local* or *surface coil* size, approximately 24 cm. These 24 cc local coils allowed for imaging of one small section of the spine at a time. Some systems offer a Buckey apparatus to allow for easy repositioning of surface coils in the area of the spine that was to be imaged.
- *Multiple-array coils* or *phased-array coils* have facilitated MR imaging of the complete spine because they allow for large FOV imaging by employing a four-coil array. This method allows for a high SNR and high-resolution images of the entire spinal cord from C1 through the conus, which occurs usually around T12 or L1.

Landmarking for Spine Imaging

For most spine imaging sequences, patients are positioned such that they are centered to the spine coil. At this time, landmark is established and is sent to the isocenter of the magnet.

- For spine imaging, the longitudinal (right to left) landmark is along the mid-sagittal plane of the patient (down the middle of the patient and along the sternal notch, xyphoid, or belly button, depending on which portion of the spine is being imaged).

- The coronal (anterior to posterior) landmark is in the middle of the neck (for cervical spine imaging) the thorax (for thoracic spine imaging) and the abdomen (for lumbar spine imaging).

- The axial (superior to inferior) landmark varies with the portion of the spine being imaged. For cervical spine imaging, the landmark is at the level of C3-C4 or at the level of the angle of the mandible or at the Adam's apple. For thoracic spine imaging, the landmark is approximately at the manubrium or approximately the level of the nipple line. For lumbar spine imaging, the landmark is at the level of the crest, approximately at the navel.

Options for Spine Imaging

Several artifacts can commonly appear on spine images. Artifacts to expect in and around the spine are *motion artifacts* from blood flow, respiration, and patient motion. A number of techniques that compensate for motion can be employed to minimize the effects of motion on image quality. These techniques include saturation pulses, cardiac gating, gradient moment nulling, and swapping of phase and frequency encoding directions. In addition, oversampling techniques minimize aliasing artifacts.

- One technique to minimize artifacts in spine imaging is to apply *presaturation pulses* both outside and within the FOV. For flow coming into the image, saturation pulses can be placed superior and inferior to imaging slices.

- To reduce motion artifacts for structures within the FOV, saturation pulses can be placed anterior to the spine. The localizer image (upper left) has no saturation pulse and the T1 spin echo (SE) image (upper center) has a saturation pulse located anterior to the spinal column.

- Electrocardiogram (ECG) leads or a peripheral gating device can be placed on patient to employ cardiac gating techniques. ECG leads can be used for spine imaging to decrease pulsatile flow motion artifacts caused by cardiac, arterial, and CSF flow near the spinal cord. *Whenever surface coils are used, especially with cardiac gating leads, it is critical to avoid creating conductive loops within the imager to avoid antenna effects* and subsequent burn injuries.
- Gradient moment nulling can be used to minimize flow motion artifact from slow flow within the FOV, such as venous and CSF flow.
- Swapping the direction of phase and frequency (SPF) encoding gradients can move motion artifacts out of the way of the anatomy (or abnormalities) to be imaged.
- Antialiasing or oversampling techniques can be used to alleviate aliasing or wrap around, especially when SPF techniques are used.

INDICATIONS FOR CONTRAST AGENTS FOR SPINE IMAGING

To gain both pathologic and anatomic information, sagittal or axial T1-weighted, short TR-TE series scanned through areas of interest can be acquired with the introduction of MR contrast agents. Intravenous contrast agents can be used to enhance lesions within the spine or spinal cord. Gadolinium is generally the contrast agent of choice for evaluating spinal lesions and lesions of the cord.

Standard Dose and Administration for Gadolinium

Gadolinium chelate has been approved by the Food and Drug Administration (FDA) for use as a contrast agent in MRI. It is recommended that gadolinium chelate be administered intravenously over several minutes followed by a 5 cc saline flush.

- Standard dose for gadolinium is 0.1 mmole/kg of body weight.
- This translates to a dose of 0.2 cc/kg.
- This translates to a dose of approximately 0.1 cc/lb or 10 cc for a 100 pound patient.

Mechanism of Action and Effects of Gadolinium on Spine Images

Gadolinium shortens the T1 and T2 times of tissues near the area that the contrast resides. The major use of gadolinium chelate involves the identification and characterization of lesions in the central nervous system CNS, such as the spinal cord lesions, as well as bony lesions in the vertebral bodies and scar tissue in postoperative lumbar disks.

- One of the important features of gadolinium chelate is that it does not cross the blood-brain barrier (BBB). Because of this feature, gadolinium chelate does not affect the relaxation times of gray and white matter within the spinal cord; the normal cord will not enhance. Lesions cause a breakdown in the BBB and will enhance.

- Gadolinium will enhance lesions within the vertebral bodies. When contrast is used for bone lesions, sequences should include fat-suppression techniques since enhanced bone lesions will otherwise become isointense with fatty marrow and become virtually invisible.

- For patients who have had surgery to correct for disk herniations and have recurrent pain, contrast-enhanced lumbar images will help differentiate between recurrent disk and scar tissue. Scar enhances but, at first, disk will not. However, after approximately 20 minutes, the disk will enhance. For this reason, timing is critical for these studies.

Cervical Spine Imaging

When evaluating a patient for cervical spine abnormalities, a surface coil is placed under the neck. Cervical spine abnormalities include disk disease, tumors, multiple sclerosis, plaques, syrinx, and Arnold-Chiari malformation, among other lesions (Figure 4-3). Arnold-Chiari malformation is a herniation of the cerebellar tonsils that is often associated with a fluid-filled cavity of the cord known as a *syrinx*. Centering for this particular lesion should be at the cervicocranial junction.

Thoracic Spine Imaging

When evaluating a patient for thoracic spine abnormalities, the coil is placed under the back between C7 and L1. Markers

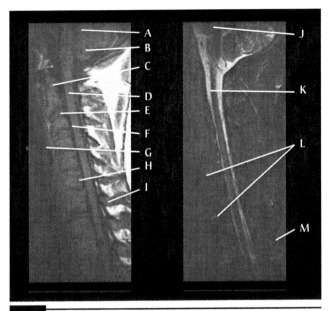

Figure 4-3 Cervical spine anatomy demonstrated in the sagittal plane. Note the anatomic locations annotated on the sagittal view of the cervical spine. *A,* fourth ventricle; *B,* cerebellar tonsils; *C,* dens; *D,* spinal cord; *E,* intervertebral disk; *F,* cerebrospinal fluid; *G,* trachea; *H,* C6; *I,* spinous process; *J,* pons; *K,* spinal cord; *L,* nucleus pulposis; *M,* spinous process.

placed along the spine help in localizing thoracic levels. When phased-array coils are used, center from C1 to L1. Large FOV localizers can be acquired to count vertebral levels, thus smaller FOV (high-resolution) images can reveal anatomy and abnormalities. Localization is especially important for the evaluation of cord compression or other lesions whereby surgeons will need to operate or center treatment on the exact level of the lesion. For patients with bowel or bladder dysfunction, there is a suggestion of lesions of the conus medullaris (located at the bottom of the spinal cord, approximately T12 to L1). For this lesion, centering should be at the level of the thoracolumbar junction.

Lumbar Spine Imaging

When evaluating a patient for lumbar abnormalities, surface coils can be placed under the lower back. Lumbar spine MR is generally acquired for disk disease (Figure 4-4). For the evalu-

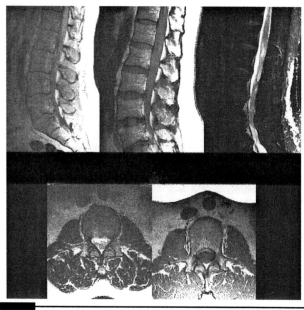

Figure 4-4 **Lumbar spine protocol.** This series represents a typical spine imaging sequence. In this series, the sagittal GE localizer *(upper left)*, sagittal SE PD *(upper middle)*, sagittal T2 FSE *(upper right)*, axial T2 FSE *(lower left)*, and T1 SE postgadolinium *(lower right)* are demonstrated.

ation of disk disease, oblique and axial views can be acquired directly through the intervertebral disk (Figures 4-5 and 4-6). For patients who have had disk surgery, intravenous contrast can help to differentiate between recurrent disk and postoperative scar.

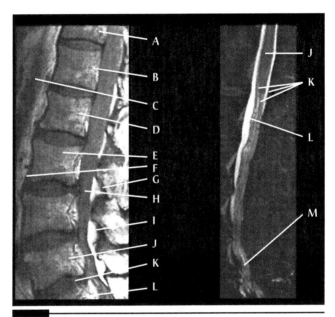

Figure 4-5 **Sagittal lumbar spine anatomy.** *A,* T12; *B,* basivertebral vein; *C,* aorta; *D,* L2; *E,* L3; *F,* anterior longitudinal ligament; *G,* ligamentum flavum; *H,* posterior longitudinal ligament; *I,* epidural fat; *J,* spinous process; *K,* L5; *L,* L5/S1 intervertebral disk; *M,* S1, *N,* conus medularis, *O,* cauda equina, *P,* cerebrospinal fluid, *Q,* nerve roots..

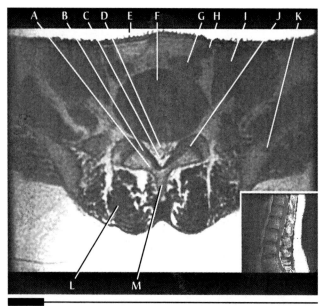

Figure 4-6 Axial lumbar spine anatomy. *A*, lamina; *B*, ligamentum flavum; *C*, epidural fat; *D*, caudal sac; *E*, subcutaneous fat (aliased or wrapped around from the back); *F*, disk; *G*, iliac vein; *H*, iliac artery; *I*, psoas muscle; *J*, facet joint; *K*, ilium; *L*, spinal muscles; *M*, spinous process.

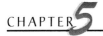

CHAPTER 5

Musculoskeletal
Imaging Procedures

Chapter at a glance

Introduction to Musculoskeletal Magnetic Resonance Imaging

Because of its high soft-tissue contrast, magnetic resonance imaging (MRI) is rapidly becoming the modality of choice to image the musculoskeletal (MSK) system for the evaluation of lesions such as tumors, degenerative changes, or posttraumatic lesions. When imaging the MSK system, however, it is not only the muscle and fat that are of interest, but also tendons, ligaments, and fibrous tissue. Ligamentous structures and cortical bone have limited mobile water protons and usually appear dark on MR images. However, although fibrous tissues appear low in signal intensity on MR images, they are nonetheless easily visualized compared with the high signal of fat and muscle. The high signal intensity shown on T1-weighted images from fat border the low signal intensity from ligaments. For this reason, ligament tears can be noted as discontinuous bands on MR images.

Furthermore, the general conception was that MR was not the modality of choice for imaging bone. However, the large bones of the joints are easily visualized on MR since marrow within the bone contains fat and water. Cortical bone, conversely, provides low signal on MRI since the water protons are too tightly bound to be influenced by the MR process. However, cortical bone can be visualized since it is adjacent to fat and muscle. The relatively high signal from muscle allows for low signal intensity of cortical bone to be visualized. Disruptions in cortical bone and, subsequently, marrow can indicate possible fractures or other lesions within the bone.

Standard Protocols for Imaging the Musculoskeletal System

Pulse sequence parameters (appropriate to evaluate joints of the body and possible lesions properly) and imaging options (to enable virtually artifact free-images of the MSK system) are selected based on anatomy and suggested abnormalities of the joints. As with other diagnostic imaging modalities, one view (set of images) is not sufficient to evaluate patients in MRI adequately. Generally, T1- and T2-weighted images are acquired in several imaging planes for optimal imaging of the MSK system. For this reason, a series of imaging acquisitions, known as a protocol, is selected for each patient to be studied with MRI.

Imaging Planes for Musculoskeletal Imaging

For most MSK imaging, all three imaging planes are required to evaluate the small structures in and around the joints.

■ Unfortunately, however, most of the joints are not oriented in orthogonal planes. For this reason, obliques are selected to observe the joint in the coronal, sagittal, and axial plane that is sagittal, coronal, or axial to the joint.

■ To avoid choosing oblique sections, in some cases the patient can be positioned in an oblique orientation. For example, for the evaluation of the anterior cruciate ligament of the knee, a sagittal oblique can be prescribed or the patient's knee can be positioned with a 15-degree external rotation.

Image Contrast for Musculoskeletal Imaging

Typically, T1-weighted images are used primarily to evaluate anatomy since they provide high signal-to-noise ratio (SNR), and T2-weighted images are used to evaluate abnormalities because of their high intrinsic contrast. For MSK imaging, the proton density (PD) images can provide high SNR images for anatomy and high signal from fluid for abnormalities.

■ T1-weighted images can be obtained in at least two imaging planes to best demonstrate anatomy. Fast gradient echo (GE), T1, or fast spin echo (FSE) T1 images can, in many cases, replace standard spin echo (SE) T1 images and offer time savings to imaging sequences.

■ Furthermore, for MSK imaging, at least one PD- and T2-weighted series should be acquired to show either tumor or fluid surrounding possible injuries.

■ Many of the T2-weighted images shown in this section are acquired with conventional SE sequences because it has been suggested that subtle findings can be missed in the blurring of FSE acquisitions.

■ Many facilities choose to replace conventional T2 SE sequences with T2 FSE sequences to save time in MSK protocols. Other facilities stay with conventional SE since blurring can occur on FSE acquisitions. At this time, it appears that approximately one half of all imaging sites in the United States have chosen FSE imaging of the joints.

Additional Musculoskeletal Sequences

In addition to providing rapid imaging sequences, GE acquisitions provide unique contrast characteristics that can be useful for MSK imaging. These characteristics include high signal from cartilage, chemical shift artifact, and high signal from flowing blood. In addition, short TI inversion recovery (STIR) sequences are commonly used as additional sequences for the evaluation of the joints.

- In most SE imaging sequences, cartilage yields low signal intensity, some GE acquisitions with high flip angles can make cartilage appear bright. By making cartilage appear bright adjacent to cortical bone, disruptions in the cartilage and tears (partial and complete) can be visualized using MRI.

- Three-dimensional GE sequences can be acquired for high resolution and reformats in additional imaging planes.

- Chemical shift imaging, in-phase–out-of-phase, or Dixon techniques can be used to demonstrate avascular necrosis (AVN). With out-of-phase imaging techniques, TE (time to the echo) images are selected such that fat and water are out of phase. The imaging results are such that signals from these areas, where fat and water are within the same voxel, will cancel. Therefore areas of fat-water interfaces become outlined by low signal. An example of out-of-phase imaging (abdomen) can be found later in this section.

- STIR sequences with TI times (the time between the inverting pulse and the excitation pulse) of approximately 150 ms (at 1.5 T) can be used to suppress the fat in the bone marrow and, as a result, allow the visualization of bone contusions.

Options for Musculoskeletal Imaging

As with MRI of other body parts, artifact compensation is required for imaging the MSK system. Artifacts such as aliasing, susceptibility, and motion can degrade MR images of the joints and render them undiagnostic.

- In small field-of-view (FOV) imaging, aliasing can be a problem when the FOV is smaller than the size of the anatomy or of the radio frequency (RF) coil being used. For this reason, antialiasing or oversampling techniques can be employed.

- In many cases, the joint of interest cannot be centered to isocenter. In these cases, off-center FOV techniques are required for high-resolution imaging of the MSK system. Off-center techniques are available on many MR imagers.

- For patients who have had previous surgeries for joint problems, metal implants can yield large metal (susceptibility) artifacts. These artifacts can be reduced by using SE or FSE sequences.

- Flow motion can cause artifacts in and around joints. In particular, for knee imaging, flow-motion artifact from the popliteal artery streak across the knee joint. To minimize this effect, saturation pulses can be employed superior and inferior to the FOV when imaging the extremities.

- In some cases, changing the direction of the phase and frequency encoding can move this artifact out of the way. This technique is known as swapping phase and frequency.

- To exploit the difference between the frequencies of fat and water, a technique known as chemical shift selective suppression (fatsat) can be used. In this technique, the frequency of water is identified and the system locates the signal from fat. The fatsat technique uses an RF pulse (at the frequency of fat) to suppress the signal from fat.

General Pathologic Conditions for Musculoskeletal Imaging

Most traumatic lesions of the joints are associated with an accumulation of fluid.

- Fluid-filled areas will appear bright on T2-weighted images or STIR images.

- In general, since tendons are expected to be low in signal intensity, any increase in signal intensity on T1-weighted images may indicate a condition known as tendonitis or tendonopathy. When signal intensity on T1-weighted images increases and persists on T2-

weighted images but does not get brighter in an intact tendon, this may present a normal finding. However, when signal intensity increases on T1-weighted images and gets brighter on T2-weighted images, it is suspected that this condition would indicate tendonitis.

PATIENT SET-UP AND POSITIONING FOR MUSCULOSKELETAL IMAGING

Positioning for MSK imaging is determined by the joint that is to be imaged. Generally, the patient is positioned supine with the joint positioned within the selected coil. Pads are placed around the patient for comfort. It is also recommended that all patients be given earplugs or headphones to minimize the effects of gradient noise.

- Patient immobilization is also important when imaging small joints. When imaging in a small FOV, such as 8 cm, patient motion of only 2 cm will move anatomy 25% out of the FOV.
- In addition, small joints such as the hand or the foot generally tend to twitch slightly. For this reason, not only proper centering, but also immobilization should be considered. *One warning: if sandbags are to be used for immobilization, it is critical to be certain to test the sandbag for MR compatibility.* Some sandbags are filled with steel shot that is, in fact, ferromagnetic. Therefore sandbags should be carefully tested to ensure their safe use in the magnetic field environment.
- Pads can be placed under the elbows or under the knees to ensure that patients do not rub the inside of the bore of the magnet.

Patient Screening for Musculoskeletal Imaging
All patients should be screened to avoid contraindications for MRI.

- Patient preparation for imaging of the lower extremity should consist of thorough screening for possible metal implants to avoid incompatible metallic implants from entering the scan room.
- All contraindications for MR apply to MSK imaging, including ferrous intracranial vascular clips, cardiac

pacemaker, and intraocular ferrous foreign bodies. These contraindications apply *unless* the patient is imaged within a small MSK imager. *Some* (not all) of these imagers have extremely small fringe fields, and since the joint (and not the entire patient) enters the magnet, these contraindications may not apply. *As always*, before proceeding with MSK imaging, avoid severe problems in the MR environment by double-checking compatibility.

■ For MSK imaging, patients who have had surgeries may have metal implants or appliances that could be problematic for MRI. In these cases, the appliance (or implant, if possible) should be tested for MR compatibility. Although metal pins and screws from orthopedic surgeries can be MR-compatible, they can produce artifacts when in the area that is to be imaged. At the least, the radiologist should be notified of the presence of the metal since the metal artifact can mimic a lesion.

■ In addition, screening for history can allow for the proper imaging of sequences to be selected. Screening for patient history and previous surgery will be helpful to ensure proper selection of protocols for imaging of the extremities. Some symptoms include pain, tenderness, rotary instability, crepitus with motion, or limited mobility.

Coil Selection and Positioning for Musculoskeletal Imaging

Imaging of the MSK system offers challenges not yet discussed in previous MRI techniques.

■ Imaging small joint spaces requires high resolution, thus patient positioning and coil selection are probably more important than in imaging studies for MR. Because imaging the MSK system requires high-resolution techniques, small, closely coupled RF coils should be used to evaluate the joints properly. In general, the smaller the coil or the better it fits the anatomy or the more closely coupled the coil is, the better the SNR. Therefore coil size should match the size of the joint being imaged in MR.

■ Small RF coils provide the signal required to use small FOV, high matrix, and thin sections required for high-resolution imaging. Many RF coils used for joint imaging are receive-only coils. However, some coils transmit and receive MR signals.

Indications for Contrast for Musculoskeletal Imaging

To gain both pathologic and anatomic information, an axial T1-weighted, short TR-TE series scanned through areas of interest can be acquired following the injection of contrast agents. In this case, gadolinium is the paramagnetic contrast of choice for MSK imaging.

- Intravenous (IV) gadolinium can be used to demonstrate inflammatory arthritis or neoplasms. In these cases, IV gadolinium is administered at the recommended dose.
- Although gadolinium has not been approved by the U.S. Food and Drug Administration (FDA) for intraarticular injection, many facilities routinely perform MR arthrography. In this technique, gadolinium is injected into the joint space to outline ligamentous structures. In most cases, gadolinium is injected into the joint space under fluoroscopic control. The patient is then brought into the MR department for imaging of the joint of interest.
- For an example of MR arthrography, see the section involving the hip.

Standard Dose and Administration for Gadolinium

Gadolinium chelate has been approved by the FDA for use as a contrast agent in MRI. It is recommended that gadolinium be administered intravenously over several minutes, followed by a 5 cc saline flush.

- Standard dose for gadolinium is 0.1 mmol/kg of body weight.
- This translates to a dose of 0.2 cc/kg.
- This translates to a dose of approximately 0.1 cc/lb or 10 cc for a 100 lb patient.
- Although it is not on the package insert as an indication for administration of gadolinium, it has been given routinely by the intraarticular method at a concentration of 1:100 and a dose of approximately 2 to 3 cc.

Magnetic Resonance Imaging of the Temporomandibular Joint

Imaging of the temporomandibular joint (TMJ) is generally acquired for the evaluation of internal derangement, TMJ syndrome, or pain. In this case, images are generally acquired to evaluate the anatomy of the joint space and the meniscus within the joint (Figure 5-1). In addition, since symptoms generally occur in patients as they open and close the mouth, T1 SE images are acquired during closed- and opened-mouth positions.

Standard Protocol Tips for Temporomandibular Joint

For TMJ imaging, patients are positioned supine with a small local coil placed over the joint.

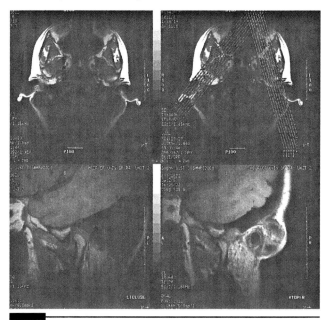

Figure 5-1 Temporomandibular joint protocol. In this typical TMJ imaging sequence, the axial GE localizer *(upper left)*, axial GE localizer with oblique acquisition slice locations *(upper right)*, sagittal oblique SE T1 with mouth closed *(lower left)*, and sagittal oblique SE T1 with mouth opened *(lower right)* are demonstrated.

■ To image these small joints of the face, local surface coils should be positioned over the joint (or joints if bilateral imaging is required) of interest.

■ Images can be acquired bilaterally when dual surface coils and multiple oblique techniques are available.

■ Images are acquired sagittal to the mandibular condyle. This plane is at an oblique to the body. The oblique is chosen from the axial and runs perpendicular to long axis of the mandibular condyle (see Figure 5-1, *upper right*).

■ Coronal obliques are acquired perpendicular to the sagittals or perpendicular to the long axis of the condyle on the axial localizer.

■ In addition, to evaluate range of motion of the joint, the patient is instructed to open his or her mouth for one sagittal oblique acquisition. Generally, obliques are acquired twice–once with the mouth closed and once with the mouth opened (see Figure 5-1, *bottom images*).

Magnetic Resonance Imaging of the Upper Extremities

There are a number of ways to evaluate the joints of the upper body for lesions. Imaging of the upper extremities before the introduction of MRI consisted of plain-film radiographs and dye-injected arthrograms. Orthopedic surgeons also performed arthroscopy, placing an arthroscope into the joint space to evaluate the anatomy of the shoulder, elbow, and wrist. In many cases, MRI replaced more invasive procedures such as radiography, arthrography, and arthroscopy because of its higher sensitivity and specificity. In addition to being noninvasive, MRI has high soft-tissue contrast and allows for high-resolution and multiplanar imaging of the upper extremities (Figure 5-2).

■ With the exception of neoplasms, the majority of lesions found in these areas are caused by insult or injury. Upper extremity injuries can be caused by a number of mechanisms, including chronic microtrauma, vascular impairment, and acute injury.

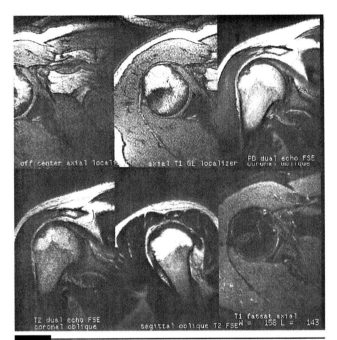

Figure 5-2 **Shoulder protocol.** In this typical shoulder imaging
sequence, the miss-centered axial GE localizer *(upper
left)*, properly centered axial GE localizer *(upper middle)*, coronal oblique dual echo PD *(upper right)*, coronal oblique dual echo T2 *(lower left)*, oblique sagittal
T2 FSE *(lower middle)*, and axial T1 fatsat *(lower right)*
are demonstrated.

- SE pulse sequences and fast-scanning techniques have
  been used to visualize soft tissues and bony structures
  better. For this reason, evaluation of the joint space, tendons, ligaments, musculature, and even bony structures
  can be visualized with MRI of the shoulder, elbow, and
  wrist.
- This section will provide an overview of upper extremity
  MRI for the evaluation of shoulder, elbow, and wrist
  lesions, such as tumors, degenerative changes, or posttraumatic lesions.

Positioning for Upper Extremities

Except for tiny patients and children, the shoulder, elbow, or wrist of interest cannot be centered to the isocenter in small-bore (56 to 60 cm) imagers. For this reason, off-center FOV techniques are required for high-resolution imaging of the upper extremities. To use off-center techniques, a large FOV coronal localizer of the chest can be acquired to localize the shoulder, elbow, or wrist of interest.

Standard Protocol for Shoulder Imaging

Positioning and coil selection for shoulder imaging may vary with the suggested abnormalities (Table 5-1) (Figures 5-3 and 5-4).

- For example, when a patient is suspected of having a bony tumor in or around the shoulder, body coil imaging could be used as a screening tool to evaluate the extent of the lesion.
- Conversely, when small ligament tears or cartilage tears are suspected, small coil, high-resolution images of that area would be optimal. Coils should be placed such that the B1 field produced from the coil is located at right

TABLE 5-1	**Shoulder Imaging Overview**	
ABNORMALITIES OF THE SHOULDER	POSITIONING FOR THE SHOULDER	ANATOMY OF THE SHOULDER
■ Impingement syndrome (degenerative changes, bursal inflammation, tendonitis) ■ Osseous changes (spurs acromion, RCT) ■ Instability (gleno-humeral joint post, multidirectional) ■ Labral tears (IGL tear, dislocation) ■ Calcific tendonitis (rotator cuff) ■ Arthritis (gleno-humeral joint)	■ Orientation–supine, head first ■ Patient–arm at side, 15-degree internal rotation to tighten tendons of rotator cuff ■ RF coil–small curved coil over shoulder ■ Landmark–over humeral head in superoinferior and anteroposterior directions ■ Off-center imaging to side of interest	■ Humeral head, scapula, clavicle ■ Glenoid labrum (glenoid fossa of the scapula) ■ Glenohumeral ligaments (inferior, superior, medial) ■ Rotator cuff (supra-spinatus and infra-spinatus teres minor, subscapularis) ■ AC joint (coraco-acromial ligament, subacromial bursa)

AC, Acromioclavicular; *IGL,* _____; *RCT,* _____; *RF,* radio frequency.

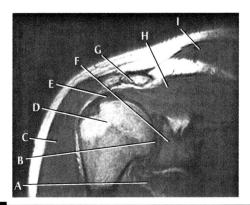

Figure 5-3 Shoulder anatomy demonstrated in the coronal oblique plane (acquired from the axial either perpendicular to the glenoid fossa or parallel to the supraspinatus muscle and tendon). *A,* infraspinatus muscle; *B,* glenoid fossa; *C,* deltoid muscle; *D,* humeral head; *E,* rotator cuff (made up of the supraspinatus tendon, infraspinatus tendon, teres minor tendon, and subscapularis tendon); *F,* scapula; *G,* acromion; *H,* supraspinous muscle; *I,* trapezius muscle.

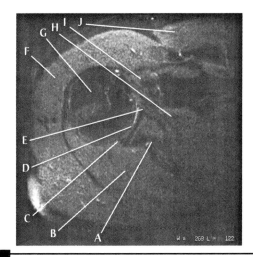

Figure 5-4 Shoulder anatomy demonstrated in the axial plane. *A,* spine of the scapula; *B,* infraspinatus muscle; *C,* posterior horn of the glenoid labrum; *D,* glenoid fossa; *E,* anterior horn of the glenoid labrum; *F,* deltoid muscle; *G,* humeral head; *H,* subscapularis muscle; *I,* coronoid process; *J,* pectoralis muscle.

angles to the main magnetic field. Therefore most coils should remain flat inside the magnet, either under or on top of the patient for optimal use of these coils.

■ Coil positioning and immobilization is critical such that the coil does not slip off the shoulder. Some coils have been designed specifically for shoulder imaging and are curved; thus they can lay over the shoulder and be snugly placed over the humeral head.

■ Patients with large muscular shoulders may present a problem for upper extremity examinations, especially in high field imagers whereby 56 to 60 cm diameter bore prohibits large patients from being imaged. In these cases, creative positioning may help to complete the examinations. In several institutions, it has been suggested that a modified swimmer's position may allow patients with large upper bodies to fit within small-bore imagers.

Standard Protocol for Elbow Imaging

Positioning and coil selection for elbow imaging may vary with the suggested abnormalities (Table 5-2) (Figure 5-5).

■ Patients are generally positioned supine in the magnet with the surface coil (firm or flexible) affixed securely to the elbow.

TABLE 5-2   Elbow Imaging Overview

ABNORMALITIES OF THE ELBOW	POSITIONING FOR THE ELBOW	ANATOMY OF THE ELBOW
■ Occult radial head fractures ■ Capitellar osteochondritis (children) ■ Osteochondritis dissecans (adults) ■ Tears of distal biceps tendon ■ Ligamentous trauma ■ Cubital tunnel disorders ■ Synovial disorders	■ Orientation—supine, head first ■ Patient—arm at side, extended ■ RF coil—whatever fits on elbow ■ Landmark— olecranon process in superoinferior and anteroposterior directions ■ Off-center imaging to side of interest	■ Humerus (trochlea and capitellum) ■ Ulna (trochlear notch, olecranon, and coronoid process) ■ Radius (radial head) ■ Radioulnar joint (annular ligament) ■ Humeroulnar and humeroradial joints ■ Medial and lateral collateral ligaments

RF, Radio frequency.

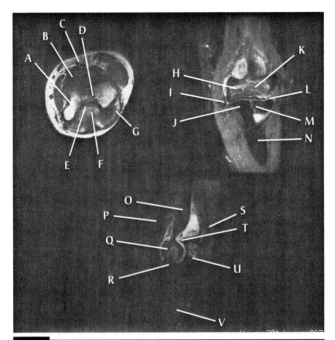

Figure 5-5 Elbow anatomy is demonstrated in the axial (upper left), coronal oblique (upper right), and sagittal (bottom) planes. *A*, capitellum; *B*, biceps brachii muscle; *C*, flexors; *D*, trochlea; *E*, olecranon fossa; *F*, olecranon process; *G*, extensor tendons; *H*, capitellum; *I*, lateral collateral ligament; *J*, head of radius; *K*, trochlea; *L*, humeroulnar joint; *M*, radioulnar joint; *N*, ulna; *O*, humerus; *P*, biceps brachii muscle; *Q*, trochlea; *R*, coronoid; *S*, triceps muscle; *T*, olecranon fossa; *U*, olecranon process; *V*, ulna.

- Pads can be placed under the elbows or under the knees to ensure that patients do not rub the inside of the bore of the magnet.
- Large patients with broad shoulders may have difficulty entering small-bore, high-field imaging systems. These patients may ask to be imaged on an *open* magnetic imager.
- Another tip is to position large patients with either one or both arms over the head.

Standard Protocol for Wrist Imaging

To gain high-resolution images of the wrist, detected wrist coils may be the best choice for wrist imaging (Figure 5-6) (Table 5-3).

- Some facilities use a dedicated wrist coil to provide the high signal required for high-resolution wrist imaging.
- Patients can be positioned supine with wrist beside the patient or in the "superman" position with arms over the head and the wrist in the isocenter. The latter can be more uncomfortable for patients with imperfect shoulder joints.

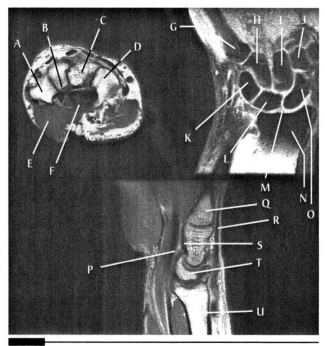

Figure 5-6 Wrist anatomy demonstrated in the axial *(upper left)*, coronal *(upper right)*, and sagittal *(bottom)* planes. *A*, trapezium; *B*, trapezoid; *C*, capitate; *D*, hammate; *E*, muscle; *F*, carpal tunnel; *G*, proximal phalanx; *H*, hammate; *I*, capitate; *J*, trapezoid; *K*, triquetruim; *L*, lunate; *M*, triangulofibrocartilage complex; *N*, radius; *O*, scaphoid; *P*, flexors; *Q*, proximal phalanx; *R*, extensors; *S*, capitate; *T*, scaphoid; *U*, radius.

TABLE 5-3	**Wrist Imaging Overview**	
ABNORMALITIES OF THE WRIST	POSITIONING FOR THE WRIST	ANATOMY OF THE WRIST
■ Carpal tunnel syndrome ■ TFCC tear ■ Trauma and fracture ■ AVN ■ Arthritis	■ Orientation–supine, feet first; or prone, head first ■ Patient–immobilized; neutral position; arm at side and extended, if supine; arm over head, if prone ■ RF coil–small; transmit and receive or receive only ■ Landmark–over ulnar styloid in superoinferior and anteroposterior directions ■ Off-center imaging to side of interest	■ Distal radius and ulna ■ Proximal carpal row (scaphoid, lunate, triquetrium, pisiform) ■ Distal carpal row (trapezium, trapezoid, capitate, hammate) ■ Radiocarpal and radioulnar joints (TFCC) ■ Ligaments (extrinsic and intrinsic) ■ Tendons (palm flexors and dorsum extensors)

AVN, Avascular necrosis; *RF,* radio frequency; *TFCC,* triangular fibrocartilage complex.

MAGNETIC RESONANCE IMAGING OF THE LOWER EXTREMITIES

Before the advent of MRI, imaging of the lower extremities consisted of plain-film radiographs and dye-injected arthrograms. Orthopedic surgeons also performed arthroscopy, placing an arthroscope into the joint space to evaluate the anatomy of the hip, knee, and ankle. In addition to being noninvasive, MRI has high soft-tissue contrast and allows for high-resolution, multiplanar imaging of the lower extremities. Because of its high sensitivity and specificity, MRI has replaced, almost entirely, more invasive procedures such as angiography, arthrography, and arthroscopy for the evaluation of the lower extremities.

■ As in the case of injuries to the upper extremities, lower extremity injuries can be caused by a number of mechanisms, including chronic micro trauma, vascular impairment, and acute injury. In the lower extremity, acute injuries include sudden contraction, forced flexion, hypertension, or overrotation.

- SE pulse sequences and fast-scanning techniques have been used to better visualize soft tissues and bony structures. For this reason, evaluation of the joint space, tendons, ligaments, musculature, and even bony structures can be visualized on MRI of the hip, knee, and ankle.

- This section will provide an overview of lower extremity imaging in MR for the evaluation of hip, knee, and ankle for lesions such as tumors, degenerative changes, or posttraumatic lesions.

Positioning for Lower Extremities

Patients are positioned supine in the magnet with the surface coil placed securely on the joint.

- When large lesions are suspected, the body coil imaging should be used as a screening tool to determine the extent of the lesion.

- For high-resolution imaging, surface coils provide the SNR to be traded for resolution.

- Generally, large patients are not a problem in lower extremity imaging since the entire patient may not need to enter the bore entirely.

Standard Protocol for Hip Imaging

Positioning and coil selection for hip imaging may vary with the suggested abnormalities (Table 5-4). Patients are positioned supine in the magnet and (when surface coils are used) the surface coil (or phased-array coils) should be placed securely over the hips.

- When a patient is suspected of having a bony tumor in or around the hip, body coil imaging could be used as a screening tool to evaluate the extent of the lesion. Conversely, when small ligament tears or cartilage tears are suspected, small-coil, high-resolution images of that area would be optimal. For the hip, some facilities recommend body coil imaging and some prefer surface coils. Finally, phased-array volume coils can be placed anterior and posterior to the hips.

- For hip imaging, slices can be acquired from above the joint to the greater trochanter and are used to evaluate the femoral head, acetabulum, and musculature of the hip. Coronals are acquired through the femoral head,

TABLE 5-4	Hip Imaging Overview	
ABNORMALITIES OF THE HIP	POSITIONING FOR THE HIP	ANATOMY OF THE HIP
■ AVN ■ Arthritis ■ Infection ■ Neoplasia ■ Osteonecrosis ■ Trauma, fracture and dislocation	■ Orientation–supine, feet first ■ Patient–legs straight or feet internally rotated ■ RF coil–body coil bilaterally hips; receive only unilateral hip ■ Landmark–over the hip joint, midway between ASIS and symphysis pubis	■ Femoral head ■ Acetabulum (ball and socket joint) ■ Ligamentum teres (acetabular fossa) ■ Innominate bone (ilium, ischium, pubic bone) ■ fibrous capsule (ilio-femoral, pubofemoral, ischeofemoral ligaments)

ASIS, Anterior superior iliac spine; *AVN,* avascular necrosis; *RF,* radio frequency; *TFCC,* triangulofibrocartilage complex.

displaying the acetabular labrum, hip joint space, sub-chondral acetabular, and femoral marrow. In the hip, the direct sagittal oblique is acquired from the medial aspect of joint to the greater trochanter. Sagittals provide a view of the ilium, anterior superior iliac spine (ASIS), acetabular roof, and femoral head articular cartilage.

Magnetic Resonance Arthrography of the Hip

To evaluate the glenoid fossa and the glenoid labrum of the hip, MR arthrography may be required (Figure 5-7).

- For this procedure, a dilute (1:100) gadolinium solution can be introduced into the hip joint, which is generally performed under fluoroscopic guidance. In this case, a small amount of iodinated contrast agent is injected in the joint space.

- When it is determined that the needle is within the joint space, the gadolinium mixture is injected. This mixture generally includes diluted gadolinium, long-acting local anesthetic, and possibly a corticosteroid. The local anesthetic makes the procedure virtually pain-free. The epinephrine allows the contrast to remain in the joint space for a longer period (for cases when the magnet may not be immediately available for imaging).

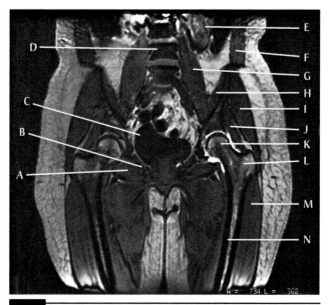

Figure 5-7 Hip anatomy demonstrated in the coronal plane.
A, obturator externus muscle; *B,* obturator internus
muscle; *C,* bladder; *D,* lumbar vertebral body; *E,* left
kidney; *F,* oblique abdominal muscles; *G,* psoas
muscle; *H,* iliac muscle; *I,* gluteus maximus; *J,* gluteus
medius; *K,* femoral head; *L,* greater trochanter;
M, quadriceps muscle; *N,* femoral shaft.

- The steroid allows for the reduction of pain in the joint.
  In this case, when the diagnostic study is normal and the
  pain is relieved, the problem involves the joint.
  Conversely, when the study is normal and the pain is not
  relieved, another source may be the cause of the problem. For this reason, a diagnostic or therapeutic study
  can help diagnose the patient.
- Subsequent to injection, the patient is imaged in multiple imaging planes with T1 acquisitions with fatsat.

Standard Protocol for Knee Imaging

For imaging the knee, patients are positioned supine and the
extremity coil is recommended (Table 5-5).

- Most extremity coils are of a volume configuration such
  that the anatomy of interest fits within the coil.

TABLE 5-5   Knee Imaging Overview

ABNORMALITIES OF THE KNEE	POSITIONING FOR THE KNEE	ANATOMY OF THE KNEE
■ AVN	■ Orientation– supine, feet first	■ Femur (medial and lateral epicondyles)
■ Arthritis		■ Tibia (tibial plateau)
■ Infection	■ Patient–foot externally rotated 10-15 degrees	■ Ligamentum teres
■ Neoplasia		■ Fibula
■ Internal derangement	■ RF coil–volume, transmit and receive coil	■ Patella (patellar endontritis)
■ Meniscal, ACL, PCL tears		■ Ligaments–medial and lateral collateral, ACL, PCL
■ Trauma, fracture and dislocation	■ Landmark–over the patella	■ Tendons (patellar)
		■ Meniscus

ACL, Anterior cruciate ligament; *AVN,* avascular necrosis; *PCL,* posterior cruciate ligament; *RF,* radio frequency.

■ For the knee, the leg is extended and placed in the coil with approximately 15-degree external rotation. This configuration will allow for a direct sagittal view of the knee to include the anterior cruciate ligament (ACL). (If this oblique positioning is not possible, oblique sections should be acquired.)

Additional Views and Options for Knee Imaging

For knee imaging, multiple obliques and additional photographic techniques can help for the visualization of structures within the knee joint (Figures 5-8 through 5-11).

■ Several ways demonstrate the cruciate ligaments in the knee and other structures that lie obliquely within the body. One technique is known as radial oblique imaging. With radial imaging, multiple obliques are prescribed from one single axial localizer. These obliques are in regular degrees of obliquity from straight sagittal, through coronal for 360 degrees, and back to sagittal. The result is a number of images in varying degrees of obliquity.

■ Photography for the visualization of the meniscus can involve wide-window techniques. With this technique, images are filmed with extremely wide window settings (bright, with many shades of gray) such that everything appears white with the exception of gray signal within the meniscus. This can, in some cases, allow for the visualization of meniscal tears.

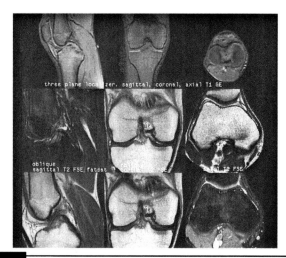

Figure 5-8 Knee protocol. In this typical knee imaging sequence, the axial GE localizer *(upper left)*, sagittal GE localizer *(upper middle)*, coronal GE localizer *(upper right)*, sagittal T2 FSE fatsat *(middle left)*, oblique coronal T2 FSE *(middle center)*, axial T2 FSE *(middle right)*, sagittal PD SE *(lower left)*, coronal PD SE *(lower center)*, and axial T1 GE fatsat *(lower right)* are demonstrated.

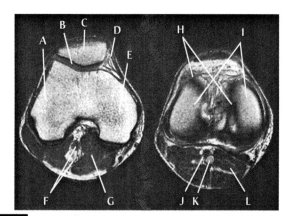

Figure 5-9 Knee anatomy is demonstrated in the axial plane. *A,* lateral epicondyle; *B,* patellofemoral joint; *C,* patella; *D,* medial retinaculum; *E,* medial epicondyle; *F,* popliteal artery and vein; *G,* gastrocnemius muscle; *H,* medial and lateral menisci; *I,* medial and lateral epicondyles; *J,* popliteal artery; *K,* popliteal vein; *L,* gastrocnemius muscle.

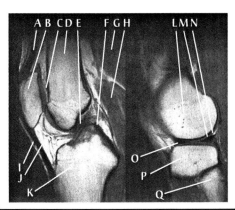

Figure 5-10 Knee anatomy is demonstrated in the sagittal (or sagittal oblique) plane. *A,* quadriceps tendon; *B,* patella; *C,* patellofemoral joint; *D,* femur; *E,* ACL; *F,* PCL; *G,* hamstring muscle; *H,* gastrocnemius muscle; *I,* patellar ligament; *J,* infrapatellar fat pad; *K,* tibia; *L,* lateral epicondyle; *M,* cartilage; *N,* posterior horn of the lateral meniscus; *O,* anterior horn of the lateral meniscus; *P,* tibia; *Q,* fibula.

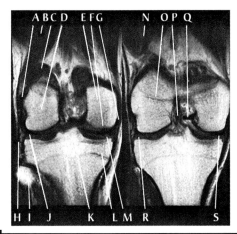

Figure 5-11 Knee anatomy demonstrated in the coronal (or coronal oblique) plane. *A,* lateral collateral ligament; *B,* hamstring muscle; *C,* gastrocnemius muscle; *D,* lateral epicondyle; *E,* medial epicondyle; *F,* cartilage; *G,* medial collateral ligament; *H,* lateral collateral ligament; *I,* fibula; *J,* lateral meniscus; *K,* tibial spine; *L,* tibial plateau; *M,* medial meniscus; *N,* quadriceps muscle; *O,* epiphyseal plate; *P,* ACL; *Q,* PCL; *R,* lateral meniscus; *S,* medial meniscus.

Standard Protocol for Ankle Imaging

For ankle imaging, patients are positioned supine with the ankle in the extremity coil (Table 5-6).

■ To evaluate the ankle with MRI, the patient is positioned with the leg straight and the foot positioned (toes up) in the extremity coil.

■ For ankle imaging, axial slices can be acquired from superior to the malleoli through the calcaneus or tibiotalar joint and can be used to evaluate the Achilles tendon. (Axial to the ankle is the same as axial to the rest of the body. However, if these images are continued through the foot, this would be considered coronal to the plane of the foot.)

■ Coronal images are acquired from anterior talus through the Achilles tendon. Sagittal images can be acquired to evaluate the long axis of tendons crossing the joint. *If the patient's foot is not positioned straight up, coronal obliques should be acquired.* (Remember, coronal to the ankle is the same as coronal to the rest of the body. However, if these images are continued through the foot, this would be considered axial to the plane of the foot.)

TABLE 5-6	Ankle and Foot Imaging Overview	
ABNORMALITIES OF THE ANKLE	POSITIONING FOR THE ANKLE AND FOOT	ANATOMY OF THE ANKLE
■ Transchondral fractures (osteochondritis, talar dome fracture, osteochondral fracture) ■ Tendon injuries (Achilles rupture, peroneal rupture, tenosynovitis) ■ Ligament injuries (sprains) ■ Tarsal tunnel syndrome ■ Foot fractures ■ Plantar fasciitis	■ Orientation—supine, feet first ■ Patient—foot pronated for foot imaging and neutral or partial plantar flexion of ankle ■ RF coil—volume, transmit and receive coil unilaterally, or head coil bilaterally ■ Landmark—over malleolus for ankle (foot, including toes)	■ Tibia ■ Fibula ■ Distal tibiofibular joint ■ Tibiotalar or ankle joint (hinge joint) ■ Ligaments (deltoid and lateral) ■ Tarsal joints ■ Tendons (Achilles)

ACL, Anterior cruciate ligament; *PCL,* posterior cruciate ligament; *RF,* radio frequency.

- Sagittal can be acquired from medial through lateral malleoli and can evaluate the tibiotalar joint, peroneal brevis, and longus tendons. *If the patient's foot is not positioned straight up, sagittal obliques should be acquired* (Figure 5-12).

Standard Protocol for Foot Imaging

To evaluate the foot with MRI, the patient is positioned supine with the foot centered in the extremity coil (see Table 5-6).

- To evaluate the foot (dissimilar to the ankle), the patient is positioned with the knee bent and the foot positioned toes-down in the extremity coil.

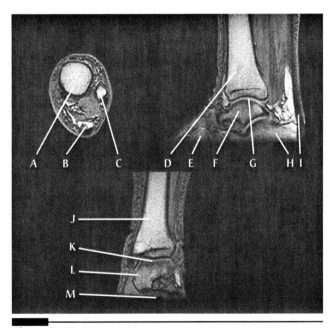

Figure 5-12 Ankle anatomy demonstrated in the axial plane. Note the anatomic locations annotated on the axial image of the ankle. *A,* tibia; *B,* Achilles tendon; *C,* fibula; *D,* tibia; *E,* proximal phalanx; *F,* talus; *G,* tibiotalar joint; *H,* calcaneus; *I,* Achilles tendon; *J,* tibia; *K,* tibiotalar joint; *L,* talus; *M,* proximal phalanx.

- For kinematic imaging of the foot, inversion and eversion can be evaluated in the coronal plane; plantar and dorsal flexion can be evaluated in the sagittal plane.
- Images acquired axial to the foot can be acquired for tarsal tunnel. (Axial to the plane of the foot—when continued posterior—would be considered coronal to the ankle.
- Images acquired coronal to the plane of the foot can be used to evaluate the metatarsals.

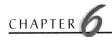
Thorax Imaging Procedures

Chapter at a glance

INTRODUCTION TO THORAX MAGNETIC RESONANCE IMAGING

To evaluate the chest for abnormalities, clinicians would prefer to visualize the airway, great vessels, brachial plexus, lungs, heart, and the mediastinum through noninvasive means. Although plain film radiography remains as the most cost-effective means for screening chest lesions, it offers low resolution and low soft-tissue contrast. Computed tomography (CT) can provide high resolution for imaging the chest, but without iodinated contrast, offers less than ideal soft-tissue contrast. Because the quality of magnetic resonance imaging (MRI) is adversely affected by motion, MRI can be difficult when used to image the thorax. However, with motion compensation techniques such as rapid imaging, cardiac gating, respiratory compensation, and saturation pulses, MRI can provide high-contrast images of thoracic structures. In addition, MRI has the capability of imaging in multiple imaging planes in two-dimensional and three-dimensional sections. This feature makes MRI ideal for imaging the chest, wherein structures lie obliquely and not in orthogonal planes. Furthermore, MRI can produce contrast differences between stationary tissues and flowing blood. Therefore dissimilar to CT, there is often no need to administer contrast agents to evaluate the heart or great vessels of the chest. However, with the administration of gadolinium, some conditions can be further evaluated for pathologic and vascular information, as well as functional information. This section will discuss imaging strategies for MR imaging of the thorax.

Standard Protocols for Imaging the Thorax

Pulse sequence parameters (appropriate to evaluate thorax and possible lesions properly) and imaging options (to enable virtually artifact-free images of the chest) are selected based on the anatomy and suggested abnormalities of the thorax. As with other diagnostic imaging modalities, one view (i.e., one set of images) is not sufficient to evaluate patients in MRI adequately. Generally, T1- and T2-weighted images are acquired in several imaging planes for optimal imaging of the thorax. For this reason, a series of imaging acquisitions, known as a *protocol*, is selected for each patient to be studied with MRI.

Imaging Planes for Thorax Imaging
For thorax imaging, the selected imaging planes (views) are chosen to display the anatomy and suggested abnormalities within the chest properly.

- For thoracic imaging, a coronal localizer image is useful to evaluate many of the structures of the chest. These structures include the lungs, trachea, heart, and mediastinum.
- Axial imaging planes are also useful for the evaluation of the same structures and act as a compliment for CT scans.
- To evaluate the "candy-cane" shape of the aortic arch, the sagittal plane is optimal.

Additional Views for Cardiac Imaging

Because the heart lies obliquely in the thoracic cavity, optimal cardiac images are obtained in oblique planes. For the heart, this includes short-axis (axial to the plane of the heart), two-chamber views (sagittal to the plane of the heart), and four-chamber views (coronal to the plane of the heart). The acquisition of these views can be problematic.

- *For the short axis view,* the coronal localizer view can provide location selections. The first location is chosen at the base of the heart at the level of the aortic root. The next location is chosen anterior at the level of the apex of the heart. Scans are acquired perpendicular to the location choices previously mentioned and a short-axis view is acquired.
- *For the two- and four-chamber views,* locations can be selected from the short-axis view. The two-chamber view is acquired with slices parallel to the interventricular septum. The four-chamber view is acquired with slices perpendicular to the interventricular septum.

Image Contrast for Thorax Imaging

Typically, T1-weighted images are used primarily to evaluate anatomy because they provide a high signal-to-noise ratio (SNR), and T2-weighted images are used to evaluate abnormalities because of their high intrinsic contrast. A number of pulse sequences can be used to evaluate the thorax, which can include spin echo (SE), fast spin echo (FSE), gradient echo (GE), and fast gradient echo or echo planar (EPI). With appropriate parameter selections, most of these imaging techniques can be acquired for T1, T2, or T2* information. In general, T1 images are acquired for evaluating anatomy and T2 images are acquired for evaluating abnormalities. T2* or gradient echo images are acquired as fast scans with high signal from flowing blood.

- For thoracic imaging, a coronal localizer image is useful to evaluate many of the structures of the chest. Generally, the localizer is acquired for T1 information with either SE (short TR-TE) or spoiled GE (short TR-TE and large flip angle). SE sequences provide a better SNR but are acquired in scan times on the order of several minutes. GE sequences provide a lower SNR but can be acquired in a breath-hold.

- For thoracic abnormalities, T2 information can be acquired with SE (long TR-TE and long imaging time), FSE (long TR-TE, long echo train length [ETL], and short imaging time), GE (short TR-TE and short flip angle in a breath-hold), or EPI (acquired in milliseconds).

- As part of the thoracic evaluation, vascular structures should also be visualized. Remember, when SE is used, flowing blood is black. These images can be referred to as *black blood images*. (*Note that on Figure 6-1 of this section, the flowing blood in the heart of the SE images is black.*)

- When GE is used, flowing blood will be bright. These images can be referred to as *bright blood images*. (*Note that on Figure 6-1 of this section, the flowing blood in the heart of the GE images is bright.*) However, susceptibility artifacts are more apparent on GE images. (*Note that on Figure 6-1 of this section on the sagittal GE localizer, there are two susceptibility artifacts on the anterior chest wall caused by the metal component of the ECG leads.*)

- In addition to conventional imaging techniques, vascular structures can be evaluated with MR angiography (MRA) techniques. MRA techniques include time of flight (TOF), phase contrast (PC), and contrast-enhanced MRA.

Additional Imaging Sequences for Cardiac Imaging

In addition to the classic cardiac imaging techniques, there are new advances, including spatial modulation of magnetization (SPAMM), perfusion and multiphase imaging.

- SPAMM modulates the magnetization thus creating a saturation effect on the image. This effect can be observed on the image as a cross-hatching of stripes. This tech-

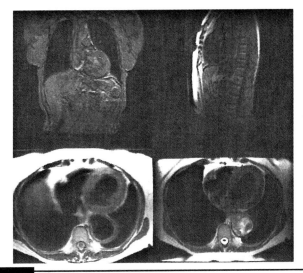

Figure 6-1 **Thorax protocol.** In this typical chest imaging sequence, the coronal T1 GEI localizer *(upper left)*, sagittal T1 GEI localizer (upper right), axial T1 FSE *(lower left)*, and axial T2 FSE *(lower right)* are demonstrated. Generally, a GE acquisition would be acquired (with or without contrast) to evaluate flow (GE images are not shown). On the axial images, we see the left ventricle of the heart as having a thick myocardial wall and the right ventricle as having a thinner wall and more anteriorly located.

nique is used in association with a multislice, multiphase acquisition. In some lesions, the persistence of stripes on images and their motion relative to cardiac and vascular motion helps to classify the lesion.

- ❏ In normal hearts, the stripes will move along with the cardiac muscle.
- ❏ In cases of myocardial infarction, the infarcted area does not contract with the normal muscle thus allowing for easy identification of the infarcted area of the heart.
- ■ Furthermore, cardiac function can be evaluated with the use of multiphase or cardiac cine.
- ■ Finally, cardiac perfusion can be evaluated with dynamic images of the heart during contrast enhancement.

Patient Set-Up and Positioning for Thorax Imaging

Patient positioning is dependent on individual patient conditions. However, for chest imaging, patients are usually positioned supine and can be positioned to enter the imager feet first. Cushions placed under the knees will increase patient comfort, an important consideration for any long procedure. Arms can be positioned over the head to minimize aliasing artifacts.

- Because of the *gradient noise* that occurs during MR procedures, it is recommended that all patients be given headphones or earplugs to wear during the examination. Earplugs can attenuate 10 to 20 db of acoustic noise that will bring the imager noise to well below the acceptable limit recommended by the U.S. Food and Drug Administration (FDA). This is even more important for thoracic imaging whereby rapid-imaging, ultra-fast, and cine techniques (which are known to be significantly louder than other imaging techniques) are often used to alleviate the adverse effects of motion on MR images.

- For thorax imaging, electrocardiogram (ECG) leads should be placed on the patient for cardiac gating. By placing ECG leads on the patient, the cardiac cycle of the patient can be monitored and used to compensate for cardiac motion.
    - ❏ Leads can be placed on the back, left axilla, or on the anterior chest. The leads must be MRI-compatible and in good condition.
    - ❏ Failure to observe safety precautions when using ECG leads can result in severe burns.
    - ❏ Care must be taken to shave any hair from the skin where leads are to be placed to ensure good ECG-skin contact.
    - ❏ An ECG skin preparation lotion or a vigorous alcohol rub will improve lead-skin conductivity. Cartilage is an excellent conductor.
    - ❏ Proper skin preparation and lead placement are fundamental to quality chest imaging.

Special Considerations for Cardiac Patients

Magnet-hemodynamic effects occur as flowing blood moves across the magnetic field. The result of this effect is an increase in the T-wave noted on the cardiac monitor. An increased T-wave is not artifactual, but rather, a real effect of the magnetic field. Generally, this elevation is not clinically significant unless the patient has compromised cardiac function. In this case, the patient should be closely monitored by pulse oxymetry. This elevation can cause degradation of image quality when cardiac gating is employed since gating techniques trigger pulse sequences from the R-wave. In cases whereby the T-wave elevation is large enough to compromise image quality, the patient can be switched to a head-first position (to try to reduce T-wave elevation) or rescheduled for another day (when the effect may not be as noticeable).

Patient Screening for Thorax Imaging

As with any MR examination, the technologist should always screen the patient for other possible contraindicated implants such as aneurysm clips in the brain, temperature-sensing Foley catheters, cochlear implants, and foreign objects in the eyes, to name a few. Patient screening is always essential in MRI. However, there are patients (such as patients with cardiac conditions) who pose a higher risk of having implanted metal or electronic devices.

- Patients with ferromagnetic metallic implants or electronic devices (e.g., *cardiac pacemakers*) should not enter the MR environment. For this reason, patients who undergo MR imaging of the chest to evaluate the heart, should be screened rigorously to avoid implants such as cardiac pacemakers from entering the scan room.
- In addition to cardiac pacemakers, temporary or old-permanent *pacer wires* can also pose significant risk to patients since induced voltages in pacer wires can, in many cases, compromise cardiac function. Therefore even when the pacemaker has been removed, pacemaker wires are often left in the chest. Recent studies in which patients with pacer wires who have been imaged inadvertently with MRI suggest that imaging these

patients pose a *relative* contraindication, rather than an *absolute* contraindication. However, before patients with pacer wires are imaged with MRI, they must meet the guidelines of these studies and proper procedure must be followed. In these cases, the radiologist should be involved in consulting with the referring physician.

■ Furthermore, the patient should be notified of all potential risks and should complete an informed consent form.

■ Sternal wires from thoracotomy and many *heart valves* are considered safe for MRI because, although the valve does move slightly in the magnetic field, its motion is no different than the motion caused by the heart.

■ *As always, it is recommended that compatibility with MRI be determined before patients with implants enter the MR scan room.*

Coil Selection and Positioning for Thorax Imaging

Radio frequency (RF) coil selection varies with the anatomy being imaged.

■ When large field-of-view (FOV) imaging is required, as in chest imaging, the body coil can be selected. Unfortunately, body-coil imaging offers a low SNR thus high-resolution imaging is usually impossible with a body coil.

■ The phased-array, transmit-receive, quadrature coil selection offers significant improvement in the SNR that can be traded for spatial resolution as compared with the body coil and receive-only surface coil. Therefore in most cases, a phased-array, transmit-receive, quadrature coil (torso coil) is used for imaging the aorta, great vessels, and the heart.

■ Phased-array coils are also designed for breast imaging. These coils are placed on the lateral and medial aspect of the breast.

■ In addition, local surface coils may be placed off-centered on the chest (for brachial plexus imaging), on the breast, or on the site of superficial lesions, when a small FOV is desired.

■ Coil selection should be based on the anatomy being scanned.

Landmarking for Thorax Imaging

Patients are centered with respect to the table and to the coil that is being used for the procedure. Landmark varies with the area to be imaged.

- For imaging the chest, the longitudinal landmark should run along the midsagittal line of the patient, the coronal landmark in the middle of the chest (midway between the anterior and posterior chest), and the axial landmark is generally at the nipple line.
- For brachial plexus imaging, the sagittal landmark can be off-centered to the side of interest.
- For the breast, landmark should be centered on the breast of interest.

Options for Thorax Imaging

Generally, several artifacts appear on thorax images, including phase ghosting or motion (flowing blood, cardiac motion, respiration, cerebrospinal fluid [CSF], or patient motion), and aliasing (wrap-around or phase-wrap). These artifacts can be minimized by the following imaging options. *Artifact compensation* techniques to use for chest imaging should be evaluated on a case-by-case basis.

- Aliasing can be reduced with oversampling techniques.
- To reduce flow motion artifacts, apply saturation pulsed inferior to the FOV to aid in the reduction of artifacts caused by flow coming into the FOV.
- Gradient moment nulling (GMN) or flow compensation (FC) can be used on SE and GE acquisitions to aid in the reduction of flow motion artifacts caused by slower flow found within the FOV. However, GMN will produce bright vessels and, in doing so, may enhance phase ghosting around the vessels.
- Since cardiac motion is always present, cardiac (pulsatile) motion compensation techniques should be considered for MR imaging of the chest. Pulsatile motion artifacts can be minimized by synchronizing the imaging sequence to the cardiac cycle, which is achieved by a technique known as *cardiac gating*. By placing ECG leads on the patient, the cardiac cycle of the patient can be monitored. The imaging system then uses the electrical

pulse that occurs during the R-wave, which is displayed on the monitor, to trigger the pulse sequence. Since the scan is triggered by the R-wave, the repetition time (TR) is now determined by the patient's heart rate.

■ *To calculate the TR*, the patient's heart rate must be determined. For example, if the heart rate is 60 beats per minute (BPM) and there are 60 seconds in a minute, then there will be an R-wave every second. In this case, if a scan is triggered every R-wave, then the TR is 1000 ms (1000 ms = 1 second). For a T1-weighted image of the chest, scans can be triggered every R-wave or TR = 1000 ms. For a T2-weighted image of the chest, scans can be triggered every other R-wave (2000 ms), every third R-wave (3000 ms), or every fourth R-wave (4000 ms). The use of cardiac gating on T1-weighted imaging and on T2-weighted imaging will decrease pulsatile flow motion artifacts created by the heart and the great vessels in the chest. This type of cardiac imaging is known as *single-phase imaging*.

Additional Options for Cardiac Imaging

Several imaging acquisitions can be acquired to evaluate the heart, including single and multiphase imaging of the heart.

■ For single-phase imaging, each phase encoding step for each image is acquired at the same phase of the cardiac cycle to minimize pulsatile motion artifact. Single-phase imaging is useful as a type of localizer image or one to best visualize the anatomy of the heart aorta and mediastinum. Initially, images are usually acquired in the axial plane. Sagittal, oblique sagittal, and oblique coronal imaging are commonly used to further evaluate complex structures such as the heart, mediastinum, and aortic arch. Single-phase imaging provides artifact-free images of the chest but provides little information about cardiac function.

■ A study of *cardiac function* requires several images at one location, acquired at multiple phases of the cardiac cycle. Remember, after the R-wave, the heart moves through its cycle. During systole, the heart is in its contraction phase; during diastole, the heart is in its relaxation phase. By selecting appropriate delays after the R-wave that triggers the pulse sequence, single-phase images can be acquired during the systolic or diastolic phase of the cardiac cycle. However, imaging all of the cardiac phases can be visualized by a technique known as cardiac cine or multiphase cardiac imaging. These techniques are used to evaluate cardiac motion, function, and flow.

■ In *multiphase cardiac imaging*, an SE pulse sequence is used with slices acquired at precise phases of the cardiac cycle. Multiphase imaging is acquired with prospective gating whereby images are triggered from the R-wave, as in cardiac gating. This technique can be performed with either single-slice (one slice location) or multislice (multiple slice locations) acquisition techniques. For example, in multislice imaging, when four slice locations and four cardiac phases are selected, slice location number one has been acquired in each of four phases of the cardiac cycle. The same is true for the other three slice locations. Therefore the result is four slices at each of four locations or a total of 16 slices. Each slice at one location shows a different period in the cardiac cycle and when viewed sequentially will create a movie of a beating heart. If the images from slice location number one were displayed dynamically in a multiple image cine loop, cardiac motion can be viewed to evaluate cardiac function at that level. One drawback to an imaging sequence of this type is that the imaging time increases with the number of slice locations or phases.

INDICATIONS FOR CONTRAST AGENTS FOR THORAX IMAGING

In addition to conventional imaging techniques, intravenous (IV) contrast agents such as gadolinium can be injected to enhance image contrast on T1-weighted images.

■ In the chest, a number of lesions will enhance with the use of gadolinium. Enhancing lesions include myocardial infarction, lesions in the lungs, mediastinal masses, vasculature, and perfusion.

- In addition to intravenous contrast agents, other liquid IV agents that are under investigation are tagged for cardiac imaging.

- There are also agents that are gaseous and can be used for ventilation imaging of the lungs. MRI of hyperpolarized noble gasses (e.g., xenon, helium) shows great promise for the future of pulmonary ventilation and perfusion, as well as cardiac and renal perfusion. These gases are polarized using a laser and a polarizing coil and are inhaled.

Standard Dose and Administration for Contrast Agents for Thorax Imaging

Gadolinium chelate has been approved by the FDA for use as a contrast agent in MRI. It is recommended that gadolinium be administered by IV over several minutes, followed by a 5 cc saline flush.

- Standard dose for gadolinium is 0.1 mmol/kg of body weight.

- This translates to a dose of 0.2 cc/kg.

- This translates to a dose of approximately 0.1 cc/lb or 10 cc for a 100 pound patient.

- Breath-holding, three-dimensional, fast multiplanar, spoiled GE scans (for enhanced MRA in the thorax) are acquired with a 20 to 40 cc bolus of gadolinium.

- For ventilation studies, hyperpolarized gas is inhaled. The dose will correspond to the lung volume.

Mechanism of Action and Effects of Contrast Agents on Thorax Images

- Gadolinium agents shorten T1 time, making vessels and vascular tumors bright on T1-weighted images.

- Three-dimensional, contrast-enhanced imaging allows for multiplane reconstruction of the heart, aorta, pulmonary vessels, and mediastinum. Scan times usually range from 20 to 30 seconds. Therefore these can be acquired in a breath-hold. The aorta is usually acquired in the sagittal plane with a three-quarter FOV to shorten scan time. Large FOVs (48 cm) can reveal the entire thoracic and a large portion of the aorta. Generally, pulmonary vasculature is best viewed in the coronal plane. Placing the patient's arms above their head diminishes aliasing. Following arterial phase, venous phase, and delayed three-dimensional acquisitions, axial fat-saturated, two-dimensional, fast multiplanar, spoiled GE images are usually acquired through the entire thorax.

■ When performing examinations for aortic dissection and aneurysm, these two-dimensional axial images should be continued through the renal arteries or to the end of the abnormality.

■ *To see a contrast-enhanced MRA of the chest, refer to the vascular section and Figure 9-3.*

■ Cardiac and lung perfusion scanning allows imaging of the efficiency of myocardial and pleural microvasculature. Rapid imaging techniques such as segmented k-space, fast GE, and echo planar imaging (EPI) allow early myocardial enhancement to be observed during the first 1 to 2 minutes postgadolinium injection. Regions of infarct have reduced signal intensity compared with healthy myocardial tissue.

■ When using hyperpolarized gasses (helium [He]) for the evaluation of ventilation of the lungs, healthy lung tissue, as well as the myocardium and kidneys absorbs the gas readily. Areas affected by pulmonary embolus and myocardial infarction show decreased perfusion and enable the targeting of diseased tissue without using radioactive isotopes. Because the gases have a short lifetime of hyperpolarization (3 He lifetime = 30 seconds), rapid-scanning techniques are required.

MAGNETIC RESONANCE IMAGING OF THE BREAST

The diagnostic tool most widely used to screen the breast for lesions is radiographic mammography. As a screening tool, mammography is helpful in demonstrating lesions in the breast. However, for staging, mammography has relatively low specificity of detected abnormalities. In addition, mammography offers little or no information for patients with dense breasts or with silicone implants. However, in lesions with specific radiographic characteristics, such as calcifications, mammography can reveal malignant lesions (Figure 6-2).

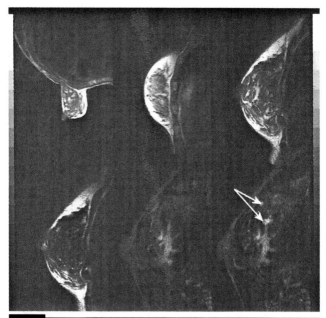

Figure 6-2 **Breast protocol (with contrast enhancement for the evaluation of lesions).** This series represents a typical breast imaging sequence. In this series, the axial local- izer *(upper left)*, sagittal localizer *(upper middle)*, sagittal high-resolution T1 SE *(upper right)*, sagittal high- resolution T2 FSE *(lower left)*, T1 3-D GE fatsat *(lower middle)*, and T1 3-D GE fatsat post-gadolinium *(lower right)* are demonstrated. Note the suspicious areas of enhancement *(arrows)* on the image.

- **MRI breast for implants:** MRI of the breast for the evalua- tion of silicone implant ruptures became popular during the class-action suit filed against manufacturers of these implants. Since mammography was suboptimal for the evaluation, MR became the modality of choice. Imaging consists of acquisition of T1 and T2 images in several imaging planes. In addition, suppression techniques help to determine whether the implant is ruptured and whether the silicone has leaked from the capsule.

- **MRI breast for lesions:** MRI, albeit sensitive to breast architecture and lesions in the breast (high sensitivity),

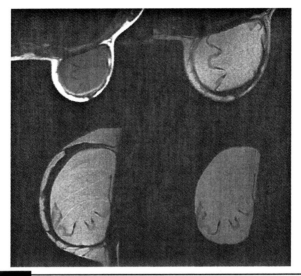

Figure 6-3 **Breast protocol for the evaluation of breast implants.** In this typical breast imaging sequence, the axial T1 GE localizer *(upper left)*, axial high-resolution T1 SE *(upper right)*, sagittal high-resolution T2 FSE *(lower left)*, and sagittal high-resolution STIR *(lower right)* are demonstrated. Note the "linguini" within the implant, which implies that the implant is likely ruptured. The "linguini" is the polyurethane bag that has collapsed and the silicone that is floating.

can be unspecific as to the cause (low specificity). This factor coupled with the higher cost and longer imaging times yields MR as an imaging modality that was, until recently, less than perfect for routine breast imaging. Improvements have been made in coil configurations, resolution, imaging times, and specialty imaging techniques that allow for more diagnostic MR images of the breast (Figure 6-3).

Imaging Planes for Breast Imaging

Frequently, high-resolution images in at least two imaging planes are acquired for breast imaging.

■ For breast imaging, the axial plane corresponds to the craniocaudal (CC) view performed during mammography

- The sagittal plane corresponds to the mediolateral oblique (MLO) view
- The coronal view is rarely acquired for breast MRI

Image Contrast for Breast Imaging

MRI of the breast can be acquired with a number of imaging strategies.

- Typical T1-weighted images are acquired with high-resolution (small FOV and thin slice thickness), SE sequences with short TR-TE combinations. Generally, these sequences take approximately 2 minutes to acquire.

- T2-weighted images should always be acquired for pathologic information, which can be achieved with long TR-TE, SE, or, for time-saving FSE acquisitions. Edge enhancement provided by long TR-TE, FSE images provides a suitable choice for detailed breast images. However, fat signal is bright on FSE images.

- High signal from fat can be nullified with fat suppression techniques in FSE images.

- Because breast studies can be somewhat lengthy, fast-scanning techniques should be considered to evaluate the breast. Another method for the acquisition of T1 information is with a sequence known as three-dimensional, spoiled gradient echo (SGE). SGE sequences can be acquired with approximately 50 ms TR times, making scan times relatively fast. These techniques should be considered when contrast agents are injected and dynamic (wash in) information is required for staging breast lesions. In addition, the three dimensions allows for higher resolution.

- For the evaluation of silicone implants, one of two options can be used to demonstrate possible leaks. These two options include silicone suppression and everything-else suppression.

  - In the case of silicone suppression, silicone is suppressed like fatsat, because silicone resonates 200 hertz (Hz) lower frequency than fat.

  - In the case of silicone imaging (i.e., everything-else suppressed), a short TI inversion recovery (STIR) sequence is used to suppress fat and water saturation is used to suppress water. In this case, only silicone is visualized (see Figure 6-2, *bottom right*).

Additional Imaging Considerations for Breast Imaging

High-resolution MRI of the breast provides high sensitivity for the detection and higher specificity for the characterization of breast lesions, not revealed on mammography or low-resolution MRI. Staging breast lesions requires high resolution to evaluate the fine detail of the borders of breast lesions.

- *High resolution* can be achieved with *small FOV, thin section, and a high-imaging matrix.*
- Because the SNR is compromised with small voxel, high-resolution images, local coils are used to buy back the reduction in the SNR.
- Another method for acquiring high-resolution, high-SNR images of the breast is with *three-dimensional volume imaging.*

Options for Breast Imaging

A number of artifacts can appear on breast images, including wrap-around or aliasing, a high signal from fat or silicone, or motion. The following are options to minimize the effects of these artifacts:

- Whenever small FOV, high-resolution imaging is employed, aliasing can occur when the FOV is smaller than the anatomy to be imaged. This is the case during breast imaging when structures of the chest wall can alias or wrap around onto the small FOV image of the breast. To minimize aliasing in breast imaging, oversampling techniques can be employed.
- Because the breast is composed largely of fatty tissue, fat suppression techniques are commonly used in breast imaging. When the high signal from fat obscures breast anatomy and subsequently abnormalities, the signal from fat can be nullified with a technique known as chemical shift selective suppression (fatsat).
- Fat suppression techniques should also be considered when contrast agents are injected to reduce the fat signal and enable better visualization of contrast enhancement.

- Other suppression techniques that can be used to allow for better visualization of breast lesions after the introduction of gadolinium include magnetization transfer techniques (MTI). MTI uses off-resonance suppression and provides better background suppression. This method, in turn, provides more obvious enhancement of breast lesions.

- Another technique for optimal fat suppression is known as spectral inversion recovery (IR). In this case, the 180-degree inversion pulse is applied only to the frequency of fat. For this reason, this technique can be used after the infusion of gadolinium.

- Fatsat can be achieved in chemicals other than fat. For cases in which breast implants are present, the signal from silicone can be suppressed. To achieve silicone suppression, the frequency of silicone must be located (100 Hz lower than fat at 1.5 T).

- Conversely, water can be suppressed with water saturation and fat can be suppressed with STIR techniques. In this case, everything *except* silicone is suppressed, thus silicone can be visualized easily.

Coil Selection and Positioning for Breast Imaging

Several coil manufacturers have developed special coils for breast imaging.

- Many of these coils are receive-only coils, some coils receive in phased-array, and several coils transmit and receive MR signals.

- RF coil selection for breast imaging is based on the size of the breast. Smaller breasts can be imaged with a small three-inch, local coil; larger breasts need either a 5-inch or a shoulder coil to accommodate breast size.

- If the coil is larger than the breast that is to be imaged, the signal and subsequently the image quality may be degraded. To compensate for improper coil filling by small breasts in larger coils, water or saline bags can be placed in or near the sensitive volume of the coil.

Patient Positioning and Set-Up for Breast Imaging

Patients positioning and comfort are always important in MRI, especially in delicate imaging techniques of the breast.

- Patients are usually positioned prone with the breast suspended pendulous (ring-type) through or in (cup-shaped) RF coils. The bra is removed and the patient gown is pulled loosely to allow the breast to hang freely in the coil. The upper abdomen and upper chest are built up with pads to allow room for the breast to hang down without obstruction from the table or pads.

- When phased-array coils are used, the breast is pressed gently between two or four coils. Coils are placed medial and lateral to the breast. Breast compression allows for a smaller volume to be imaged and a lesser number of thin (high-resolution) sections of the breast. This technique is used primarily to shorten overall imaging time. In addition, the slight compression of the breast helps to minimize artifacts caused by breast motion.

- When possible, coils are placed posterior enough to enable the visualization of the chest wall.

Indications for Contrast Agents for Breast Imaging

Contrast enhancement has helped to determine the cause of lesions but does not provide 100% accuracy for staging breast lesions. As specificity improves, MRI is expected to be used more routinely as a staging tool for breast lesions; and because MR sensitivity is high, MR will certainly be used more often for breast screening as the price and scanning times are reduced (see Figure 6-3).

- All cancers enhance with contrast in MRI. Unfortunately, some benign lesions also enhance. To distinguish benign from malignant lesions of the breast, high-resolution and rapid-imaging sequences can be acquired.

- Dynamic imaging techniques are acquired by selecting the slice of interest from previous acquisitions. Once the location is determined, a preinjection image is acquired in that area. Then, the contrast is injected. Immediately following injection, images of the selected location are acquired as rapidly as the system allows. These sequences can be played back in a multiple-image display loop to visualize dynamic wash-in of breast lesions. It is believed that lesions that enhance rapidly are likely to be malignant and that lesions that enhance slowly are likely to be benign.

■ Staging breast lesions requires high resolution to evaluate the fine detail of the borders of breast lesions. High resolution is required to evaluate the architecture of the lesion. It is believed that lesions with smooth borders are likely to be benign and lesions with speculated borders are likely to be malignant.

CHAPTER 7

Abdomen Imaging Procedures

Chapter at a glance

INTRODUCTION TO ABDOMEN MAGNETIC RESONANCE IMAGING

Historically, clinicians have chosen imaging modalities such as computerized tomography, conventional angiography, general radiography, and ultrasound to detect and evaluate many abdominal conditions and diseases. Compared with magnetic resonance imaging (MRI), these modalities were less expensive, more easily accessible, and offered more familiarity for the referring clinicians. Traditionally, the use of MRI in the abdomen has been as a problem-solving technique. The benefits of MRI high-spatial resolution, excellent soft-tissue contrast, less invasive techniques, and the use of nonionizing radiation were overshadowed by its shortcomings: cost, length of the examination, and physiologic motion artifacts. However, several recent technical advances and new imaging techniques including improvements in coil and magnet design, faster more advanced pulse sequences and new contrast agents, have improved the accuracy and utilization of abdominal MRI.

STANDARD PROTOCOLS FOR IMAGING THE ABDOMEN

Imaging of the abdomen requires T1 and T2 acquisitions, however, motion artifacts can degrade the quality of abdomen images. The advent of new, ultra-fast scanning techniques allow for breath-hold T1-, T2-, and dynamic-enhanced images of the abdomen with fewer motion artifacts. Today, the majority of imaging sequences acquired for the abdomen are rapid sequences acquired in a breath-hold. For this reason, images are, for the most part, free of artifacts. The ability to produce images without motion artifacts is directly related to the implementation of the faster generation of gradient technology. These powerful, high-performance gradient systems can produce not only breath-hold acquisitions, but also high-resolution (smaller fields of view and thinner slices) and suppressed images (chemical saturation) in less time than ever imagined. These new advancements combine to provide high-resolution, rapid-imaging protocols for imaging the abdomen.

Imaging Planes for Abdomen Imaging

For abdomen imaging, the selected imaging planes (views) are chosen to display the anatomy and suggested abnormalities within the abdomen.

- Because the anatomy of the abdomen is displayed adequately in coronal plane, coronal T1-weighted, gradient echo, *localizer* images are acquired to establish landmarks. Some imaging systems allow for a three-plane (sagittal, coronal, and axial) localizer for optimal positioning for subsequent imaging sequences.

- Following the localizer sequences, T2-weighted and proton density (PD)–weighted (FLAIR) images are generally acquired in the axial plane. Additional axial sequences are acquired with T1 gradient echo acquisitions in and out of phase or for dynamic-enhanced sequences following contrast enhancement. Axial sequences are optimal for the evaluation of the liver, kidneys, spleen, pancreas, and adrenal glands.

■ The coronal plane is used for evaluating the kidneys and the adrenal glands.

Image Contrast for Abdomen Imaging

Currently, the standard abdominal MRI includes three sequences: T1-weighted, T2-weighted, and contrast-enhanced images. Depending on the patient's condition and cooperation level, a variety of pulse sequences are available that will generate T1-weighted and T2-weighted images. Many imaging systems allow for breath-hold, gradient echo sequences for T1-weighted imaging and echo train sequences for T2-weighted imaging.

■ Although spin echo and inversion recovery sequences commonly have been used to generate T1-weighted images, the breath-hold, spoiled gradient echo sequence (SGE) is the most important and versatile pulse sequence for evaluating abdominal disease. SGE scans, coupled with the use of phased-array coils, can be used to replace longer duration scans such as the conventional spin echo and inversion recovery sequences.

❏ The advantages of SGE sequences include the reduction and in some cases the absence of breathing artifacts, true T1-weighting, and complete coverage of the abdomen in a single breath hold.

❏ In addition, the time to the echo (TE) can be altered with SGE imaging to produce in-phase and opposed-phase imaging. When fat and water protons are in-phase, their signals add; when they are opposed-phase, their signals cancel each other. This cancellation effect will produce a signal void or a black ring artifact around organs, such as the kidneys, where fat and water interfaces occur within the same voxel. On a 1.5 T magnet, a typical echo time for in-phase imaging would be approximately 4.2 ms and about 2.1 ms for opposed-phase scans. Opposed-phase imaging is an accurate and effective tool to detect and demonstrate diseased tissues. For example, common indicators for opposed-phase imaging would be fatty infiltration in the liver and lipids within adrenal masses in an effort to characterize them as benign adenomas. To see out-of-phase images refer to Figure 7-1 *(upper center and upper right)*.

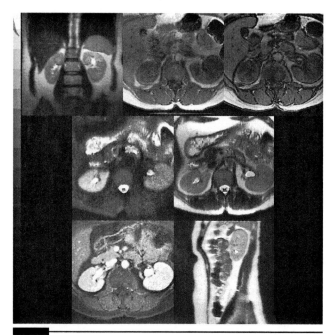

Figure 7-1 Abdomen protocol. In this typical abdomen imaging sequence for the evaluation of the kidneys, the coronal localizer SSFSE *(upper left)*, axial T1 GE in phase *(upper middle)*, axial T1 GE out of phase *(upper right)*, T2 FSE fatsat *(middle left)*, T2 FSE *(middle right)*, post-gadolinium axial T1 *(lower left)*, and sagittal SSFSE localizer *(lower right)* are demonstrated.

- The primary goal of T2-weighted imaging is to detect increased fluid in diseased tissues, which results in high signal intensities on the images. Spin echo sequences are generally employed when performing T2-weighted imaging. The sequences can be either conventional spin echo or an echo train spin echo sequence, such as fast spin echo or turbo spin echo.
  - ❏ Conventional spin echo scans are rather lengthy sequences that are plagued by patient motion.
  - ❏ However, fast spin echo (FSE) sequences produce only slight image blurring, most notably observed on PD-weighted images. Presently, FSE sequences are used more frequently on state-of-the-art systems

because of their shorter acquisition times, increased spatial resolution, and decreased examination time. An FSE sequence reduces the scan time by performing more than one phase encoding step and subsequently filling more than one line of k-space per TR (recovery time) period. This is achieved by using an operator-controllable parameter called the echo train length, which consists of several 180-degree refocusing pulses. As each refocusing pulse is applied, an echo is produced and a different phase encoding step is performed. Short TI inversion recovery (STIR) may also be performed to acquire T2-weighted information. TI is the time between the inverting pulse and the excitation pulse.

■ When the entire image is acquired in one shot (all of k-space is filled in one TR period) a T2 image can be acquired in a breath-hold. This technique is known as single shot FSE (SSFSE). This type of image allows for heavily T2-weighted images whereby only water is bright and nearly all other structures of the abdomen are dark. These sequences are known as MR hydrography (MR water images) and are used for MR cholangiography or MR urography.

❑ The development of breathing-independent, T2-weighted sequences (SSFSE) allows the acquisition of individual image sections in as little as 225 ms, greatly reducing any motion artifact.

❑ This technique reduces imaging times, but the resulting signal-to-noise ratio (SNR) is less as a result of the partial Fourier technique that is used. SSFSE technique aptly demonstrates lesions with high fluid content such as hemangiomas and cysts. The sequence obviates motion artifacts from bowel peristalsis and respiration.

■ STIR sequences can be modified as an FSE sequence used to suppress the signal from fat.

❑ Both FSE and FSE STIR can be performed as a breath-hold scan to reduce breathing artifacts.

❑ STIR sequences use short TI times of approximately150 ms at 1.5 T.

ANATOMY AND PHYSIOLOGY OF THE ABDOMEN

To evaluate the anatomy of the abdomen, the clinician begins by defining the vasculature and following it to the viscera (Figures 7-2 and 7-3).

- Defining the vascular and visceral structures in the abdomen can begin by following the descending abdominal aorta, which is located approximately midline and anterior to the vertebral column. At the level of the first lumbar vertebrae (L1), the celiac axis arises anteriorly from the descending aorta and branches into the left gastric (to feed the stomach), hepatic (to feed the liver), and splenic (to feed the spleen) arteries. Following closely to the celiac trunk inferiorly is the superior mesenteric artery (SMA), which also arises anteriorly from the descending aorta at the lower level of L1. The

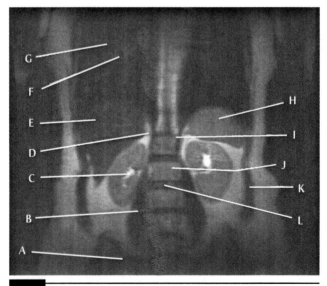

Figure 7-2 Abdomen anatomy demonstrated in the coronal plane. *A,* SI joint; *B,* psoas muscle; *C,* right kidney; *D,* right adrenal gland; *E,* liver; *F,* pulmonary vessel; *G,* lung; *H,* spleen; *I,* cruz of the diaphragm; *J,* lumbar vertebral body; *K,* oblique abdominal muscles; *L,* intervertebral disk.

SMA branches to supply the small and large intestinal tracts. Both the right and left renal arteries are positioned inferior to the SMA and extend laterally from the descending aorta. These arteries feed the kidneys bilaterally. Next, following along the abdominal aorta are the right and left gonadal arteries, which also extend laterally from the descending aorta and can be identified anterior to the psoas muscles that extend along the vertebral column. Finally, the inferior mesenteric artery (IMA) extends anteriorly and supplies blood to the remainder of the colon.

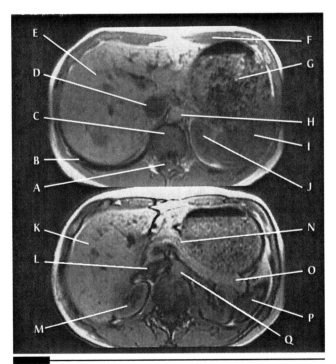

Figure 7-3 Abdomen anatomy demonstrated in the axial plane. *A,* spinal cord; *B,* lung; *C,* vertebral body; *D,* IVC; *E,* liver; *F,* abdominal muscles; *G,* stomach; *H,* aorta; *I,* spleen; *J,* left kidney; *K,* liver; *L,* IVC; *M,* right kidney; *N,* pancreas (head); *O,* pancreas (tail); *P,* spleen; *Q,* aorta.

- The inferior vena cava (IVC) is the first structure that needs to be identified in conjunction with the hepatic portal system. The IVC, which returns blood back to the right atrium, is positioned slightly midline and anterior to the vertebral body. Traveling inferior down the IVC are the three hepatic veins. The right and left hepatic veins extend laterally, whereas the middle hepatic vein branches from the IVC anteriorly. Following next is the hepatic portal vein, which is located anterior to the IVC and posterior to both the duodenum and head of the pancreas. The left renal vein can be identified at the level of the second lumbar vertebrae (L2) as it crosses over the midline to drain its contents into the IVC. As it continues across the midline, it can be observed anterior to the abdominal aorta and immediately inferior to the SMA. Next is the splenic vein, which is located anterior to the left renal vein and follows midline to join the superior mesenteric vein to form the hepatic portal vein. The inferior mesenteric vein empties into the splenic vein, and both of these structures are located posterior to the pancreatic body.

Patient Set-Up and Positioning for Abdomen Imaging

Patient positioning depends on individual patient conditions. However, for abdomen imaging, patients are usually positioned supine and can be positioned to enter the imager feet first. Cushions placed under the knees will increase patient comfort, an important consideration for any long procedure. Hearing protection should always be used when performing MRI.

Patient Screening for Abdomen Imaging

Remember, all patients should be screened to avoid contraindications for MRI.

- Contraindications include aneurysm clips, cardiac pacemakers, and intraocular foreign bodies.
- In addition, postoperative abdominal clips or intra-abdominal clips or filters may produce artifacts that can be misinterpreted in MR images.

■ For this reason, a thorough screening of family members or referring physicians may be required to avoid contraindications and misinterpretations to MR imaging.

Coil Selection and Positioning for Abdomen Imaging

Because of several new technical developments, images that demonstrate a high SNR with little or no motion artifacts are now common when imaging the abdomen.

■ One of these technical advancements has been the development and use of phased-array multicoils. Although phased-array coils are not necessarily new to MRI, they have contributed greatly to the advancement of abdominal MR image quality, particularly through improved uniformity of signal and increased SNR.

■ This technology consists of multiple coils and receivers whereby their individual signals are combined to generate images with an improved SNR while benefiting from a large field of view (FOV) displaying increased anatomical coverage.

■ The increased SNR afforded by phased-array coils allows the acquisition of smaller FOVs and thinner slices, producing higher resolution images compared with the standard body coil. For the most part, more abdominal lesions can be detected using phased-array coils compared with the body coil since SNR is better and can therefore be traded for higher resolution.

■ One drawback of phased-array technology is the high cost. This may, however, be justified by the marked improvement in overall image quality. A second disadvantage is that subcutaneous fat immediately subjacent to the coils tends to have extremely high signal intensity on non-fat-suppressed images, which can generate ghosting artifacts from motion. These marked artifacts can be reduced by using fat saturation, anterior-placed saturation bands, or breath-hold sequences.

Options for Abdomen Imaging

In the past, MR images of the abdomen were of poor quality, characterized by a low SNR and problematic motion artifacts.

- These artifacts originate from several sources including respiration, bowel peristalsis, and pulsatile flow in the heart and abdominal vessels.
- In light of these circumstances, the challenge has always been to produce high-quality images with good conspicuity of disease.
- However, conventional motion-suppression techniques can be employed to help reduce these troublesome artifacts. These techniques include respiratory compensation, abdominal binding, saturation pulses, gradient moment nulling, cardiac gating, multiple averaging (NSA), and chemically selective fat-suppression and anti-spasmodic medications.
- When used alone or in combination, these techniques can produce images relatively free of motion artifacts.

INDICATIONS FOR CONTRAST AGENTS FOR ABDOMEN IMAGING

In clinical practice, contrast is employed to improve the detection and evaluation of various diseases and conditions. Certain MRI enhancement agents affect the T1 and T2 relaxation times of different tissues, increasing a contrast difference. Today, many contrast agents are available for abdominal imaging, including T1 agents, targeted T1 agents, T2 agents, and oral and rectal agents.

T1 Contrast Agents

The T1 paramagnetic contrast agent gadolinium is most widely used for abdominal dynamic contrast enhancement.

- Paramagnetic agents cause the decreasing of T1 times, which results in brighter tissues on T1-weighted images. Peak enhancement differences occur shortly after the injection of gadolinium, and occasionally, lesions begin to enhance after only 2 minutes. Therefore rapid-scanning techniques should be employed to maximize the detection and characterization of abdominal lesions. SGE sequences acquired in a breath-hold should be used when performing dynamic-enhanced imaging.
- Since the liver, spleen, and kidneys are vascular organs, contrast enhances these structures almost immediately.

For liver, spleen, and pancreas imaging, enhanced images in the axial imaging plane best demonstrate anatomy and abnormalities. For renal imaging, enhanced images in the coronal imaging plane best demonstrate anatomy and abnormalities.

Hepatocyte-Directed Contrast Agents

Hepatocyte-directed contrast agents, which have a paramagnetic T1 shortening property, are organ-specific enhancing solutions used to further facilitate hepatic imaging.

- In addition to enhancing the liver, these agents are also excreted by the biliary system into the bile ducts and gallbladder, providing the potential for functional MR cholangiography (fMRC). Because of this characteristic, functional information such as bile transit times and ampulla and biliary duct patency can now be determined; fMRC also offers excellent anatomic evaluation of the biliary system.

- The greatest application for hepatocyte-directed agents may be the detection of metastases, not only because of differential enhancement between liver tissue and metastatic lesions, but also because the longer imaging window allows the use of high-resolution matrices that can identify tiny lesions. Persistent liver enhancement has been shown 24 hours after the initial infusion.

- Injection-related discomforts such as facial flushing are mild but frequent. The chance of a mild reaction is substantially minimized when these agents are slowly administered during a 1- to 3-minute intravenous (IV) infusion.

T2 Contrast Agents

Reticuloendothelial agents are T2-relaxation contrast agents that reduce the signal intensity of normal liver tissue.

- The Kupffer's cells within the liver will consume approximately 80% of the administered dose. Tissues that contain Kupffer's cells will have a shortening in T2 relaxation times, which results in a loss of signal intensity. However, liver tissue that does not contain Kupffer's cells does not lose signal intensity. Therefore normal liver parenchyma will appear extremely dark on T2-weighted images, and hepatic lesions will become more conspicuous because of the increase in signal intensity compared with the darkened background liver.

■ Metastases and some primary liver tumors lack Kupffer's cells and, subsequently, do not take up contrast and do not lose signal intensity. This loss of signal from normal liver tissue improves the conspicuity and delineation of hepatic lesions.

■ These agents may improve the visualization of a greater number of lesions and the segmental location of lesions. Dissimilar to gadolinium, reticuloendothelial contrast cannot be injected dynamically; rather, it requires a 30-minute IV infusion. However, this agent can be used successfully at all field strengths and does not require the MR system to generate breath-hold scans.

Oral and Rectal Enhancement Agents

Presently, oral and rectal agents are not as commonly used as intravascular agents, but this can change in the near future.

■ Oral contrast agents have been researched extensively for bowel imaging applications. Negative oral agents have been beneficial when imaging anatomic structures that are either surrounded by or in close proximity to the gastrointestinal tract. When imaging the pancreas and duodenum, some clinicians use these negative oral agents to show the delineation of the bowel on T1-weighted sequences. These agents can also be used when performing MR cholangiography to evaluate the biliary system for stenoses without any high-signal, bowel-superimposing, biliary structures such as the common bile duct and pancreatic duct.

■ In addition, negative oral agents have been instrumental in the definitive diagnosis of suspected cases of undescended testicles. Air has also been used as an effective contrast agent in the rectum. The prostate and uterus can be demonstrated more clearly when imaging the pelvis by introducing a signal-intensity void in the distended rectum.

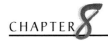
Pelvis Imaging Procedures

Chapter at a glance

INTRODUCTION TO PELVIS MAGNETIC RESONANCE IMAGING

Before the introduction of magnetic resonance imaging (MRI), imaging of the pelvis was generally limited to ultrasound (US) and computed tomography (CT). US can provide an overview of female anatomy, including the uterus and ovaries, and male anatomy, including the prostate and seminal vesicles, but with limited resolution. CT can also be used, however, with limited image contrast when acquired without oral, rectal, or intravenous (IV) contrast agents. MRI provides high soft-tissue contrast with high resolution in a noninvasive manner. However, pelvic imaging can be challenging because physiologic motion degrades image quality. Recent advances in imaging capabilities such as fast-scanning and signal-suppression techniques combined with coil technology such as surface or local coils, phased-array, or multicoil systems have made MR capable of imaging small structures within the pelvis with limited artifacts. As a result, MRI has become an alternative for the evaluation of the male and female pelvis. This section will describe MRI of the pelvis.

STANDARD PROTOCOLS FOR IMAGING THE PELVIS

For the evaluation of the pelvis for both men and women, T1 and T2 images should be acquired in multiple imaging planes. In many cases, rapid imaging sequences are chosen in an attempt to provide virtually artifact-free imaging of the pelvis. Generally, T1 images are acquired to evaluate anatomy and T2 images are needed to evaluate abnormalities. However, for the pelvis (male and female) many of the structures are better evaluated anatomically by T2-weighted images. Protocols for the male pelvis vary from female protocols depending on the abnormalities expected, but these protocols nearly always include T2-weighted images in two or more imaging planes.

PATIENT SET-UP AND POSITIONING FOR PELVIS IMAGING

Patient positioning is dependent on individual patient conditions. However, for pelvis imaging, patients are usually positioned supine and can be positioned to enter the imager feet first. Patient positioning in pelvic imaging depends on the radio frequency (RF) coil to be used and the anatomy to be imaged. For example, when the body coil is used, prone positioning can be used to minimize respiratory motion artifacts in the pelvis and lower abdomen. However, when the phased-array or endorectal coils are used, supine positioning is optimal for patient comfort. Cushions placed under the knees will increase patient comfort, an important consideration for any long procedure. Hearing protection should always be used when performing MRI.

Coil Selection and Positioning for Pelvis Imaging

Although many pelvic imaging examinations are performed with the use of the body coil, a pelvic array may be required for the evaluation of smaller pelvic structures.

- The pelvic phased-array coil can be used to provide an increased signal-to-noise ratio (SNR). Since SNR is increased with the use of the coil, a high-resolution image can be acquired with a 256 × 256 imaging matrix, 20 to 24 cm FOV, 4 to 5 mm, with 0 to 1 mm spacing for the evaluation of smaller pelvic structures.

- When an endorectal coil is used for pelvic imaging, a sagittal, large FOV, spin echo localizer is usually performed. When using high-resolution imaging techniques, it is important to ensure proper patient centering. Off-center FOV techniques are available on most systems. Therefore, when it is impossible to get the area of interest directly into the isocenter of the magnet, these techniques should be employed. Endorectal coils are inserted while the patient is in the left lateral decubitus position. After coil placement, the patient is rolled into the supine position for imaging. Patient centering is critical for high-resolution, small (as low as 8 cm) FOV imaging techniques. In addition, antispasmodics are essential for endorectal-coil imaging to minimize rectal wall motion.

Patient Screening for Pelvis Imaging

As in any MR examination, the technologist should always screen the patient for other possible contraindicated implants such as aneurysm clips in the brain, cardiac pacemaker, cochlear implants, and foreign objects in the eyes, among others. There are a few devices that are of particular concern for pelvis imaging, including:

- Women who have birth control devices such as intra-uterine devices (IUDs) or diaphragms may create artifacts for female pelvis imaging.

- Men with any one of several penile implants that may be problematic for MRI because they are ferrous and can be attracted to the magnetic field.

- For this reason, a thorough screening of patients, family members, or referring physicians may be required to avoid contraindications to MRI.

- MRI is acceptable for the pregnant woman, and many MR studies are actually required for the fetus.

Options for Pelvis Imaging

Because motion remains a problem in pelvic imaging, motion-compensation techniques such as antispasmodics, respiratory compensation, saturation pulses, and gradient moment nulling (GMN) should be used whenever possible.

- To retard peristalsis, to minimize motion artifacts from bowel motion, and to maximize comfort in patients when the endorectal coil is used, antispasmodics should be considered. Glucagon (1 mg) can be administered intramuscularly (for longer action) or intravenously (for faster action) before imaging to reduce peristaltic motion artifacts.

- In small FOV imaging, antialiasing techniques should be used to minimize wraparound artifacts along the phase and frequency encoding axes.

- In addition, since phase ghosting often occurs in pelvic imaging arising from peristalsis in the bowel, phase- and frequency-encoding directions can be manipulated (swap phase and frequency techniques) to move phase ghosting artifacts away from the anatomy of interest. By selecting phase encoding from right to left on axial, high-resolution images of the pelvis, phase ghosting artifacts will appear from right to left, across the image and away from the area of interest. This phenomenon commonly occurs in the pelvis during prostate imaging but can also occur when imaging other pelvic structures.

Indications for Contrast Agents for Pelvis Imaging

Contrast enhancement can improve the diagnostic ability or MRI. The contrast agent primarily used for pelvis imaging is gadolinium.

- For cases when dynamic information is required, fast gradient echo sequences can be performed during contrast injection. These sequences provide perfusion information in vascular pelvic structures.

- In addition, when flow information is desired, flow-sensitive, gradient echo and MRA techniques can be employed after contrast enhancement. For vascular imaging, a three-dimensional, T1 gradient echo acqui-sition is acquired during contrast injection. These angiographic techniques will be discussed in the vascu-lar section.

■ Some facilities have also used gadolinium to evaluate the colon. In these cases, gadolinium is diluted with saline and introduced into the rectum. This procedure is fol-lowed by the acquisition of a three-dimensional, T1 gra-dient echo acquisition. This acquisition can be reformat-ted and post processed for the evaluation of the colon in multiple imaging planes.

STANDARD DOSE AND ADMINISTRATION FOR GADOLINIUM

Gadolinium chelate has been approved by the U.S. Food and Drug Administration (FDA) for use as a contrast agent in MRI. It is recommended that gadolinium be administered intra-venously over several minutes, followed by a 5 cc saline flush.

■ Standard dose for gadolinium is 0.1 mmol/kg of body weight.

■ This translates to a dose of 0.2 cc/kg.

■ This translates to a dose of approximately 0.1 or 10 cc/lb for a 100 pound patient.

■ For enhanced MRA in the pelvis, breath-hold, three-dimensional, fast multiplanar spoiled gradient echo scans are acquired with a 20 to 40 cc bolus of gadolini-um.

■ Although gadolinium is not indicated for oral or rectal use, colon imaging is performed at some facilities. For colon imaging, 10 ml of gadolinium can be diluted in 100 ml of saline.

■ It should be noted that contrast is considered a precau-tion for patients who are pregnant or lactating.

STANDARD PROTOCOLS FOR FEMALE PELVIS MRI

In general, the female pelvis protocol consists of T1- and T2-weighted images in three imaging planes. Depending on the patient's condition and cooperation level, a variety of pulse sequences are available that will generate T1-weighted and T2-weighted images. However, most imaging systems will employ breath-hold gradient echo sequences for T1-weighted imaging and FSE (fast spin echo) sequences for T2-weighted imaging.

- For a localizer image in the female pelvis, the coronal plane is generally acquired.

- To evaluate the uterus (endometrium and junctional zone), T2-weighted images are acquired in the sagittal imaging plane. The sagittal plane is best for revealing the uterine anatomy. The T2 image contrast allows for the visualization of the uterus, the inner lining (junctional zone), and the innermost lining (the endometrium). On T1-weighted images, these structures appear isointense or they have the same signal intensity. However, on T2-weighted images, the endometrium has a high signal intensity, the junctional zone will be low signal intensity, and the uterus will be intermediate. These T2-weighted, FSE sequences are performed using long TR (3000 to 5000 ms), long TE (140 ms), echo train length (ETL) of 16, and echo spacing of 20 ms. (TR = repetition time and TE = the time to the echo.)

- Additional imaging sequences (both T1- and T2-weighted images) can be acquired in the axial plane to see pelvic anatomy and its relationship to other pelvic structures such as the bowel, bladder, vessels, and lymph nodes.

- The coronal plane is also useful for the evaluation of the ovaries and fallopian tubes. Since T2 contrast helps with the evaluation of the uterine and ovarian structures, T2 images are often acquired in the coronal plane.

- For patients in which cervical ectopic pregnancy or cervical cancer is suggested, oblique imaging through the cervical is also performed to further characterize this specific region.

The use of fatsat (chemical shift selective suppression) is also applied to certain imaging techniques to further characterize abnormalities observed on MRI (Figures 8-1 through 8-3).

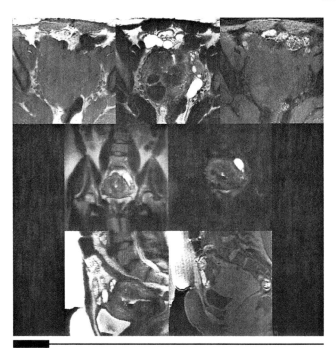

Figure 8-1 Female pelvis protocol. In this typical female pelvis imaging sequence, the axial T1 GE *(upper left)*, axial T2 FSE *(upper middle)*, axial T1 GE fatsat *(upper right)*, coronal SSFSE localizer *(middle left)*, coronal T2 FSE fatsat *(middle right)*, sagittal T2 FSE *(lower left)*, and sagittal T1 GE fatsat *(lower right)* are demonstrated. In general, the sagittal T2 image of the female pelvis best demonstrates the uterus; the coronal T2 image demonstrates the ovaries.

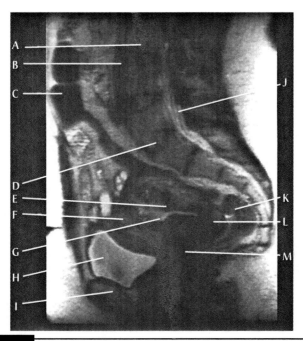

Figure 8-2 Anatomy of the female pelvis (sagittal plane). For female imaging, the sagittal plane best demonstrates the uterus. *A,* vertebral body; *B,* aorta; *C,* bowel; *D,* intervertebral disk; *E,* junctional zone of the uterus (low signal); *F,* fundus of the uterus; *G,* endometrium (high signal); *H,* urinary bladder; *I,* symphysis pubis; *J,* caudal sac; *K,* rectum; *L,* cervix; *M,* vagina.

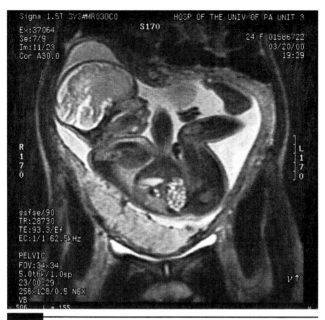

Figure 8-3 In this fetal MRI sequence, the fetus and placenta are visualized for the evaluation of both the viability of the infant and the location and quality of the other products within the uterus.

Standard Protocols for Male Pelvis MRI

A typical pelvis protocol for the evaluation of the male pelvis, particularly the prostate gland, includes a localizer, followed by high-resolution images in three imaging planes, followed by a large FOV (field-of-view) image of the abdomen and pelvis.

- Fast gradient echo sequences take approximately 1 to 2 seconds to acquire and provide a suitable localizer for coil placement and anatomic localization. However, when prostate cancer is suspected, bone metastasis may accompany the disease. In this case, spin echo, T1-weighted images can be substituted for the localizer series to provide a reasonable look at the vertebral bodies in the spine as well as localize the position of the coil.
- The next sequence acquired for the evaluation of the prostate gland includes short TR-TE, spin echo images acquired in the axial view with high-resolution imaging techniques. This small FOV acquisition is used primarily to evaluate gross anatomy of the prostate, localization of the coil relative to the prostate gland, and to screen for blood subsequent to prostate biopsy.
- Axial, sagittal, and coronal oblique high-resolution, T2, FSE sequences are performed using long TR (3000 to 5000 ms), long TE (140 ms), ETL of 16, and echo spacing of 20 ms. In cases when higher resolution is required, 8 cm FOV images with a 512×512 matrix can be acquired on imaging systems with these capabilities.
- Sagittal imaging planes allow for the visualization of the prostate gland, through which the urethra runs and the seminal vesicles are observed.
- The coronal plane demonstrates the prostate gland, the vas deferens (superior and centrally located) and the seminal vesicles (bilateral to the vas).
- T2-weighted images in the axial plane demonstrate the peripheral zone (higher signal) and the central gland (intermediate signal intensity). Superior to the prostate gland is the fluid-filled seminal vesicles (high signal intensity). An area of a high- and low-signal intensity within the central zone of the prostate gland can represent

benign prostatic hyperplasia (BPH). This enlarges the prostate gland and, on occasion, necessitates that a TURP be performed to dilate the urethra. A low signal-intensity area in the peripheral zone of the prostate gland can correspond to the blood from a biopsy or a cancerous lesion.

■ Large FOV, short TR-TE sequences, acquired through the abdomen and pelvis are performed to screen for metastatic disease in the lymph nodes and bone metastasis. Imaging sections are acquired with the body coil and large FOV. Because of the typical location of metastatic nodes, axial imaging sections can be acquired from the symphysis pubis up to the renal hila (Figures 8-4 and 8-5).

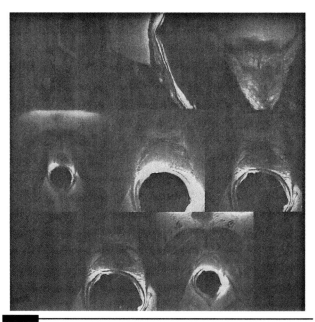

Figure 8-4 **Male pelvis protocol.** In this typical male pelvis imaging sequence, the sagittal SSFSE localizer *(upper left)*, sagittal T2 FSE *(upper middle)*, coronal T2 FSE fatsat *(upper right)*, axial SSFSE localizer *(middle left)*, axial T1 SE *(middle center)*, axial T2 FSE fatsat *(middle right)*, axial SSFSE *(lower left)*, and axial T1 GE *(lower right)* are demonstrated.

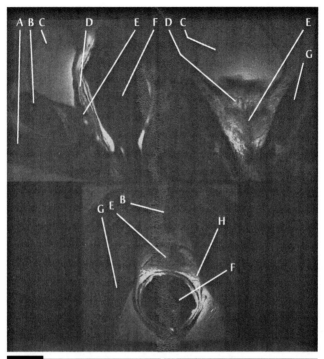

Figure 8-5 Anatomy of the male pelvis demonstrated in the sagittal, coronal, and axial planes. For the evaluation of the prostate gland, imaging in all three planes with high resolution is necessary. *A,* penis; *B,* symphysis pubis; *C,* urinary bladder; *D,* seminal vesicles; *E,* prostate gland; *F,* rectum; *G,* internal obturator muscle; *H,* neurovascular bundle.

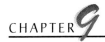

CHAPTER 9

Vascular Imaging Procedures

Chapter at a glance

INTRODUCTION TO VASCULAR MAGNETIC RESONANCE IMAGING

Magnetic resonance imaging (MRI) of the vessels has been made possible with the advent of rapid-imaging sequences and vascular motion-compensation techniques. Before the introduction of fast imaging, it was difficult to image moving structures such as blood within vessels because MR acquisition time was long relative to flow motion. Before magnetic resonance angiography (MRA), the patient would be required to undergo conventional angiography to evaluate both the morphology and hemodynamics of the neurovascular system. In this section, vascular MRI techniques will be discussed, including flow-sensitive conventional imaging techniques, MRA, and velocity encoding techniques.

FLOW IMAGING: AN OVERVIEW

In both gradient echo and spin echo imaging, vessels can be visualized. On gradient echo sequences, flowing blood appears bright. To make flow appear brighter, an option known as flow compensation or gradient moment nulling (GMN) can be applied. Most MRA techniques (time of flight [TOF], phase contrast [PC], and contrast-enhanced) are modified gradient echoes. On spin echo sequences, flowing blood appears dark. To make flowing blood appear even darker, saturation pulses can be applied in the direction of incoming blood flow. Saturation pulses not only eliminates phase ghosting artifacts, but also provide an intraluminal signal void for distinction between patient and obstructed vessels. Vascular imaging techniques will be discussed in this section.

Spin Echo Imaging

Spin echo techniques provide images whereby flowing blood appears black. Saturation pulses applied outside the field of view (FOV) saturates the blood before it enters the FOV, thus vessels appear black.

- For this reason, the vascular system can be evaluated with conventional spin echo imaging sequences and presaturation pulses. This technique is known as black blood angiography. Spin echo imaging with presaturation pulses enable the visualization of the vascular system such that flowing vessels appear black.
- Because spin echo imaging sequences provide images without distraction of susceptibility effects, black blood angiography may be a suitable choice for the evaluation of blood flowing through the vessels.
- Presaturation can be used to evaluate vascular patency. However, because presaturation uses an additional RF pulse, the specific absorption rate (SAR) is increased and some slices may be lost as a result.

Gradient Echo Imaging

The vascular system can be evaluated with gradient echo imaging. On gradient echo images, flowing blood appears bright. GMN is a first-order, velocity-compensation technique used to refocus the signals from slow moving protons (as in blood flow).

- Therefore GMN is a technique to compensate for flow motion artifacts and to enhance the signal in flowing blood. With GMN, protons from, for example, venous blood or cerebrospinal fluid (CSF), are put in phase. GMN compliments flow by making vessels containing slow flowing spins appear bright thus enhancing the blood and CSF signal.

■ Several tradeoffs for using GMN are that it requires a longer minimum time to the echo (TE) and a reduction in the available number of slices. GMN is not as effective on spin echo sequences or in areas of rapid flow such as the aorta. However, it is helpful in gradient echo MRA techniques.

MAGNETIC RESONANCE ANGIOGRAPHY: AN OVERVIEW

Conventional MRA is usually performed by one of two techniques: TOF or PC. TOF relies on flow-related enhancement. PC relies on phase shifts of moving spins.

Time of Flight Magnetic Resonance Angiography

TOF relies on flow-related enhancement (FRE) to distinguish moving spins from stationary spins.

■ Stationary spins in a slice (two-dimensional [2-D]) or slab (three-dimensional [3-D]) receive multiple RF pulses, usually with a short repetition time (approximately 28 to 50 ms) and are therefore saturated, producing little MR signal.

■ Flowing spins (blood) that receive the RF pulse or pulses flow out of the slice or slab and are replaced with fresh, fully magnetized spins. These unsaturated spins flowing into the imaging slice or slab produce a high MR signal.

■ The saturation level differences between the stationary spins (background tissue) and flowing spins (blood) contribute to the images contrast.

■ These images are then stacked and subjected to a post-processing technique to produce a projection-type image that resembles a conventional angiogram. The most commonly used projection technique is known as maximum intensity pixel (MIP).

Time of Flight Magnetic Resonance Angiography Image Contrast

In addition to the velocity of blood flow, several imaging parameters also affect saturation level differences and thus contrast. These parameters include flip angle, repetition time (TR), TE, voxel volume, slice orientation, and thickness.

■ The greater the flip angle or the lower the TR, the greater the saturation of the stationary spins and the lower the signal from the background tissues. In general, the flip angle and TR are selected based on the blood flow velocity and the acquisition technique (2-D or 3-D).

■ In general, when TE times are low, TOF MRA is improved. Low TE times allow little time for dephasing to occur thus higher signal from flowing vessels. Increased TE times also contribute to increased flow artifacts.

■ It is best to acquire MRA sequences using small voxel volumes. As the voxel volume is increased, the loss of signal from dephasing of the spins within an imaging voxel (intravoxel spin phase dispersion) also increases, which can lead to loss of signal within a vessel, although blood is flowing.

■ As previously mentioned, contrast is also dependent on blood flow velocity. The slower the blood flow, the more saturated the blood spins, and the less contrast between flowing spins and stationary spins. The velocity of the blood flow must be high enough to replace the saturated flowing spins in the slice or slab with fresh, unsaturated spins, otherwise there will be little or no contrast.

Two-Dimensional Time of Flight Magnetic Resonance Angiography

A 2-D TOF sequence is acquired using thin sequential slices and is good for viewing a large area of coverage but with lower resolution than with a 3-D sequence.

■ Generally, the slice thickness is approximately 1.5 mm.

■ To maximize the signal from flowing blood and reduce the signal from the background tissue, the TR is usually between 30 and 50 ms, and the flip angle usually ranges from 45 to 70 degrees.

■ Additionally, flow-related enhancement can be maximized for the given flow velocity by acquiring the slices perpendicular to the blood flow. Because the slices are extremely thin (1.5 mm), the blood does not have to be flowing particularly fast to flow out of the imaging slice before becoming saturated.

■ Advantages of the 2-D TOF sequence include the ability to obtain images of blood flow over a large area, such as the common carotid arteries, the pelvis, and lower extremities, with overall scan times of approximately 5 to 10 minutes, depending on the number of slices.

■ Because the slices are acquired sequentially, any motion or change in patient position during the acquisition will cause a misregistration artifact on the projection (MIP) images.

■ Another disadvantage of 2-D TOF is an artifact resulting from pulsatile flow, often referred to as the "Venetian blind" or "stair step" effect.

Three-Dimensional Time of Flight Magnetic Resonance Angiography

Acquisitions using 3-D TOF acquire a slab or volume rather than a thin 2-D slice. The volume is then encoded to create slices or partitions through the slab. This acquisition is beneficial for high resolution but provides a limited area of coverage.

■ Compared with 2-D acquisitions, 3-D acquisitions can produce images with a higher signal-to-noise ratio (SNR) and thinner slices thus higher resolution.

■ Improvements in gradient technology further enhance the ability to acquire 3-D sequences with extremely short TE times. In some instances, the TE can be less than 1 ms.

■ Using rapid 3-D acquisitions with small voxel volumes and a short TE, susceptibility artifacts, signal loss from intravoxel spin phase dispersion, and pulsatile flow artifacts are greatly reduced.

Multiple Overlapping Thin Slab Angiography

Multiple overlapping thin slab angiography (MOTSA) has advantages over both traditional 2-D TOF and 3-D TOF. This technique provides the high resolution of a 3-D acquisition with the large area of coverage of a 2-D acquisition.

- This technique involves the excitation of numerous smaller 3-D slabs that overlap each other versus the use of one thick single slab. Acquiring the data in this formation reduces the distance that the blood must travel into the imaging plane and minimizes the saturation effects of slowly moving blood.

- Better visualization of both arterial and venous blood is appreciated with MOTSA thus making it a useful diagnostic technique in many regions of the body. MOTSA has often been used in the brain, although other applications include the aortic arch, abdomen, and peripheral vasculature.

- The downside to this technique is longer acquisition times compared with using one single slab, as with 3D TOF. However, it can cover a larger region of interest similar to the coverage of a 2-D TOF acquisition.

Phase Contrast Magnetic Resonance Angiography

PC MRA uses a bipolar gradient system to provoke changes in phases of moving spins. PC MRA provides directional and velocity information but with longer scan times than TOF MRA.

- Two acquisitions acquired with gradient polarities swapped are subtracted or added to create phase contrast angiograms.

- PC MRA acquisition results in magnitude and phase images.

- Unsubtracted combination of flow-sensitized image data is known as magnitude images; the subtracted is called a phase image.

Flow Encoding Axes

To sensitize the images to flow in a given direction, gradients are employed in that direction, which allows for directional information.

■ When a bipolar gradient pulse is applied along the Z-axis, phase shifts are provoked. In this case, PC MRA is sensitized to the flow from superior to inferior.

■ To sensitize for flow in other directions, bipolar gradients can be applied in all three dimensions: X (for right to left flow), Y (for anterior to posterior flow), and Z (for superior to inferior flow). These are known as flow encoding axes.

■ As the number of flow encoding axes is increased, imaging time increases.

Velocity Encoding

In addition to sensitizing to flow direction, PC MRA can also sensitize to flow velocity, which allows for velocity information.

■ Velocity encoding (VENC) compensates for flow velocity within vessels by controlling the amplitude or strength of the bipolar gradient.

■ When the VENC is selected lower than the velocity within the vessel, aliasing can occur, producing low signal intensity in the center of the vessel but improved delineation of vessel wall.

Three-Dimensional Phase Contrast Magnetic Resonance Angiography

PC MRA can be used effectively in the evaluation of lesions with multidirectional flow such as in arteriovenous malformations, aneurysms, venous occlusions, congenital abnormalities, and traumatic intracranial vascular injuries. These sequences generally provide long imaging times.

■ As with clinical imaging, 3-D offers a high SNR and spatial resolution and the ability to reformat images in a number of imaging planes, retrospectively. 3-D volume acquisitions can be used to evaluate intracranial vasculature with 28 slices, 20-degree flip angle, TR of less than or equal to 25 ms, 1 mm slice thicknesses, VENCs of 40 to 60 cm/sec, and flow encoding in all directions. (When 60 slices are chosen, the flip angle should be reduced to 15 degrees.)

■ The disadvantage, however, is that with 3-D PC MRA, imaging time increases with the TR, NEX, the number of phase encoding steps, the number of slices, and the number of flow encoding axes selected. For this reason, scan time can approach 15 minutes, which may be an unacceptable time for uncooperative patients.

Two-Dimensional Phase Contrast Magnetic Resonance Angiography

PC MRA can be acquired with either 2-D or 3-D acquisition strategies, which generally involve shorter imaging times than with 3-D techniques.

- 2-D techniques provide flow direction information in acceptable imaging times of 1 to 3 minutes. Intracranial applications of 2-D PC MRA can be acquired with a TR of 18 to 20 ms, 20-degree flip angle, and slices of 20 to 60 mm.

- VENCs can be chosen from 20 to 30 cm/sec for venous flow, 40 to 60 cm/sec for higher velocity with some aliasing, and 60 to 80 cm/sec to determine velocity and flow direction.

- For the carotid arteries, 2-D PC MRA parameters would include 20- to 30-degree flip angles, a TR of 20 ms, and VENCs of 40 to 60 cm/sec for better morphology with aliasing and 60 to 80 cm/sec for quantitative velocity and directional information.

- When a 2-D PC MRA acquisition has been flow encoded from superior to inferior, blood flowing from the superior direction will appear white, and blood flowing from the inferior direction will appear black. In this way, flow direction can be evaluated with 2-D PC MRA.

- 2-D PC MRA acquisitions cannot be reformatted and viewed in other imaging planes.

BODY MAGNETIC RESONANCE ANGIOGRAPHY CHALLENGES

For the evaluation of the vasculature of the body, each of the previously mentioned MRA techniques should be evaluated for the optimal technique.

- PC MRA is useful for multidirectional flow but is sensitive to any motion (i.e., moving structures will appear bright on PC MRA). Because there is a great deal of motion in the abdomen (e.g., respiration, peristalsis, blood flow), PC MRA is not optimal for the evaluation of body vasculature.

■ TOF MRA is optimal when blood flow is perpendicular to the slice plane. This method becomes challenging for structures in the chest, abdomen, and pelvis. Furthermore, 3-D TOF is useful for high resolution but offers limited coverage. 2-D TOF provides larger area of coverage but lower resolution. For these reasons, conventional TOF MRA (either 2-D or 3-D) is suboptimal for the evaluation of body vasculature.

Enhanced Magnetic Resonance Angiography

To overcome the obstacles provided with conventional MRA techniques, contrast-enhanced MRA can be employed. To accomplish this task, a T1 gradient echo (modified TOF MRA) acquisition can be acquired during the injection of gadolinium contrast.

■ To achieve high-resolution MRA in this manner (for the evaluation of smaller vessels), 3-D gradient echo acquisitions can be acquired.

■ For enhanced MRA of the body, it is preferable to acquire these images in a single breath-hold to eliminate respiratory motion. A rapid 3-D acquisition with a TR of less than 10 ms can accomplish this task in as little as 30 seconds.

■ The imaging plane for optimal coverage of the abdominal and pelvic vessels is coronal plane.

■ For the aortic arch, the sagittal plane is optimal to view the "candy cane" shape of the arch.

Rapid Infusion of Intravenous Gadolinium

The saturation resulting from the in-plane flow and the extremely short TR can be overcome by a bolus intravenous (IV) injection of gadolinium.

■ The presence of gadolinium shortens the T1 relaxation of flowing blood, which increases the MR signal from the flowing blood.

■ Gadolinium can be introduced by an injection, by way of an MR-compatible power injector, or manually. Whichever method is chosen, the injection should be extremely rapid, lasting approximately 20 seconds.

- For hand injection, a 50 cc syringe is used for the gadolinium since 40 cc will be injected. The syringe is attached to the 3-way stopcock in the same direction as the extension tubing. The saline flush solution is in a 20 cc syringe oriented 90 degrees to the gadolinium syringe. It is advisable to use the same syringe configuration to avoid confusion between the gadolinium and saline syringes.
- The timing of the injection and the acquisition is critical to the success of the procedure. The exact timing will depend largely on the cardiac output of the patient. In general, if the acquisition time is between 25 and 30 seconds, then the scan can begin when half (20 cc) of the contrast agent has been injected. For longer scans (45 seconds to 1 minute), the injection and scan can begin at the same time.
- In general, the acquisition of the mid-portion of k-space (usually the middle of the acquisition) should be acquired when the concentration of gadolinium in the area of interest is at its peak.

Postprocessing Techniques for Magnetic Resonance Angiography

After completing MRA acquisitions, the raw data can then be reconstructed into projection images. Various methods can be incorporated for viewing the reconstructed MRA. These techniques include maximum projection intensity (MIP) and shaded surface display (SSD).

- MIP is a projection ray tracing technique that produces multiple projection images following data acquisition and reconstruction. This technique works by identifying the pixel intensity along each pixel in a projection image and the pixels along each ray or line along the 2-D data set. (This may be characterized as a light shining through the volume of data.) To obtain the MIP, the projection pixel is assigned the maximum pixel intensity found along the ray traversing the imaging volume. This process is repeated until a complete projection image is obtained and can be repeated for viewing in a rotation or cine loop in various projection angles or degrees.

- SSD produces a surface rendered image. (This may be characterized as a light shining onto the volume of data.) SSD provides a better 3-D view of the vascular data, though small vessels may be lost as resolution is decreased.
- Another means for the evaluation of vascular anatomy is with a technique known as segmenting, whereby each vessel can be traced and subsequently removed from the image. In this case, each vessel can be viewed individually and free from the superimposition of neighboring vessels.

Anatomy and Physiology of the Vascular System

For simplification, vascular anatomy can be divided into arteries and veins. Although capillaries connect these two vascular systems, they are not generally visualized by MR and thus will not be described in this section. As a general review, arteries carry oxygenated blood from the heart and veins carry deoxygenated blood to the heart. Imaging of the arteries and veins of the body can be achieved by a number of MRA techniques, including TOF, PC, and enhanced MRA. Vasculature and imaging techniques for each anatomic location will be discussed in this section.

Patient Positioning, Protocol, and Coil Selection for Magnetic Resonance Angiography of the Head

Vascular imaging for each anatomic location within the body should be evaluated by the vascular configuration, flow velocity, and vessel size.

- For the head, arterial blood flow velocity is high, vessel diameter is small, and direction is multidirectional. Although there is multidirectional flow, and because flow velocity is high and vessels are small, 3-D TOF is the best choice for arterial brain imaging.
- For venous flow, however, PC MRA is best.
- Patient positioning for MRA of the brain is generally similar to positioning for brain MRI. Patients are positioned supine and in a transmit-receive head coil. In fact, most MRA studies of the head begin with full-brain imaging.

■ Patient screening is always recommended to avoid contraindications, and patients should always be provided
   hearing protection.

Brain Vascular Anatomy

Vascular anatomy of the head can be evaluated by arterial and
vascular structures.

Arteries of the Brain

■ The main arterial vessels of the head are associated with
   the circle of Willis (COW). These vessels define the circulatory system for the brain.

■ The internal carotid arteries (right and left) enter the
   head bilaterally. Each internal carotid artery curves at
   the level of the pituitary gland to form a "saddle" shape
   known as the carotid siphon. Superior to that structure,
   each internal carotid artery bifurcates into the anterior
   and middle cerebral arteries (MCA). The anterior cerebral artery (ACA) feeds the frontal lobes and the MCA
   feeds the parietal lobe.

■ A small vessel that communicates between the ACAs is
   known as the anterior communicating artery. This artery
   forms the anterior portion of the COW.

■ The vertebral arteries (right and left) enter the skull
   through the foramen magnum. These two vertebral
   arteries join to form the basilar artery, which runs along
   the anterior surface of the pons.

■ Superior to this structure, these arteries bifurcate to
   form the posterior cerebral arteries (PCA). These PCAs
   supply blood to the posterior portion of the brain.

■ Two small vessels "communicate" from the internal
   carotid arteries and the PCA bilaterally. These are
   known as the posterior communicating arteries (PCOM).
   The PCA (bilaterally) and the PCOM form the posterior
   portion of the COW (Figure 9-1).

Veins of the Brain

■ Venous structures begin with the large drainage vein
   located along the longitudinal axis of the patient. This
   vein runs under the skull but on top of the brain, from
   the forehead to the middle of the back of the skull,
   known as the superior sagittal sinus.

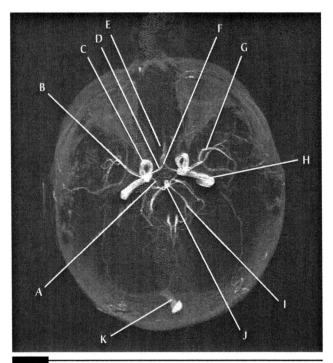

Figure 9-1 Brain vascular anatomy (mostly arterial) demonstrated in the axial plane. This axial acquisition (collapsed MIP) of the vasculature of the brain was acquired with 3-D TOF MRA. This technique is recommended for the visualization of smaller vessels. *A*, right posterior communicating artery; *B*, right middle cerebral artery; *C*, right carotid siphon; *D*, right anterior cerebral artery; *E*, right anterior cerebral artery; *F*, anterior communicating artery; *G*, left middle cerebral artery; *H*, left internal carotid artery; *I*, left posterior cerebral artery; *J*, basilar artery; *K*, superior sagittal sinus.

- Below to the superior sagittal sinus and running along the top of the corpus callosum is another drainage vein known as the inferior sagittal sinus.
- The inferior sagittal sinus drains into the straight sinus that runs in the tentorium to the confluence of sinuses.
- The superior sagittal sinus drains into the confluence of sinuses and into the transverse sinuses, and then runs

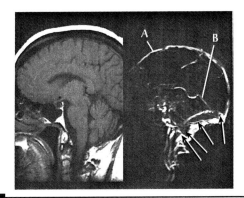

Figure 9-2 Brain vascular anatomy (venous) demonstrated in the sagittal plane. This sagittal acquisition of the vasculature of the brain was acquired with 2D PC MRA. This technique is recommended for the evaluation of venous structures of the head. *A,* superior sagittal sinus; *B,* straight sinus. The other vessels *(arrows)* beginning in the back of the head from superior to inferior include the confluence of sinuses, transverse sinus, sigmoid sinus, and internal jugular vein.

from medial to lateral on both sides of the posterior portion of the brain at the level of the cerebellum.

- The transverse sinuses drain into the sigmoid sinus, which drains into the internal jugular vein (Figure 9-2).

Typical Vascular Abnormalities of the Brain

There are a number of typical abnormalities that can be visualized by MRA of the brain.

- Arterial abnormalities include aneurysm, stroke or vascular disease, and arterovenous malformation (AVM).
- Venous abnormalities includes venous occlusion or thrombosis.

Patient Positioning, Protocol, and Coil Selection for Magnetic Resonance Angiography of the Neck

Vascular imaging for each anatomic location within the body should be evaluated according to the vascular configuration, flow velocity, and vessel size.

- For the neck, arterial blood flow velocity is high, vessel diameter is medium (not as fast as intracranial and not as slow as venous), and the flow is in one direction. For this reason, 2-D TOF is best to cover a large area of coverage.
- For the bifurcation, high resolution is better for the evaluation of small lesions. In this case, 3-D TOF may be useful for the evaluation of the carotid bifurcation. Some facilities use enhanced MRA to visualize from the aortic arch to the COW.
- Patient positioning for MRA of the neck is generally similar to positioning for neck MRI. Patients are positioned supine and a receive coil is placed over the anterior neck. In fact, most MRA studies of the neck begin with full-neck imaging.
- Remember, patient screening is always recommended to avoid contraindications, and patients should always be provided hearing protection.

Typical Vascular Abnormalities of the Neck

A number of typical abnormalities can be visualized by MRA of the neck.

- Arterial abnormalities include vascular disease, plaque, or stenosis.
- Additional abnormalities include partial or complete occlusion.

Patient Positioning, Protocol, and Coil Selection for Magnetic Resonance Angiography of the Chest

Vascular imaging for each anatomic location within the body should be evaluated according to the vascular configuration, flow velocity, and vessel size.

- For the chest, arterial blood flow velocity is high, vessel diameter is large, and the flow is multidirectional. For this reason, 3-D contrast-enhanced MRA is best to visualize thoracic vessels.
- To evaluate pulmonary vessels, the coronal plane is optimal.
- To evaluate the aortic arch (the "candy cane" view), the sagittal plane is the optimum.

- Patient positioning for MRA of the chest is generally similar to positioning for chest MRI. Patients are positioned supine in a torso-array coil or body coil. These patients generally have MRI of the chest along with the MRA study.
- Remember, patient screening is always recommended to avoid contraindications, and patients should always be provided hearing protection.

Chest Vascular Anatomy

The heart is a hollow, muscular, contractile organ that is the center of the circulatory system and provides the necessary force to circulate blood throughout the vascular system.

- The heart is composed of four chambers, each with its own specific purpose in directing blood flow through the body.
- Contraction of the heart chambers is known as systole. Diastole is the term used to describe the relaxation phase.
- The right atrium is one of the four chambers and is responsible for receiving deoxygenated blood from the superior vena cava, inferior vena cava, and the coronary sinus.
- The next chamber that takes up the majority of the anterior surface of the heart is the right ventricle. This chamber receives blood from the right atrium through the tricuspid valve.
- The pulmonary trunk branches off the right ventricle superiorly and posteriorly and then divides into the left and right pulmonary arteries. The responsibility of the pulmonary arteries is to transport blood to the lungs for oxygenation.
- The furthermost posterior chamber of the heart is the left atrium, which forms most of the base of the heart. Oxygenated blood is transported to the left atrium through the pulmonary veins that branch off the lateral walls of the left atrium.
- The last of the four chambers to be identified is the left ventricle. This chamber appears furthest to the left and can be characterized by its thick myocardial wall.

- Arising medially from the left ventricle is the ascending aorta, which arches posteriorly to the left and continues down to become the descending aorta.
- Arising from the ascending aorta are the coronary arteries, which branch off superiorly to the semilunar valve.
- The brachiocephalic, left common artery, and left subclavian arteries arise from the aortic arch anteriorly to posteriorly.
- In addition to the heart and great vessels are other thoracic structures that need to be identified during imaging because of their relationship to the other anatomic structures in the mediastinum. The trachea is located anterior to the esophagus and descends to the level of the sixth thoracic vertebrae (T-6), where it branches into the left and right pulmonary bronchi. This bifurcation is also known as the *carina*. Both the left and the right pulmonary bronchi sit posterior to their corresponding pulmonary artery.
- The esophagus is located anterior to the vertebral body and descends through the neck and superior mediastinum. It continues to lie anterior and to the right of the descending aorta in the posterior aspect of the mediastinum (Figure 9-3).

Typical Vascular Abnormalities of the Chest

When imaging the chest, abnormalities in the aorta are some of the main reasons one might consider performing an MRI or MRA for diagnosis.

- Aortic dissection is one type of abnormality that involves a tear or rip in one or several layers of the aortic wall. When a dissection occurs, blood flows through the tear, filling the space between the layers of the aorta and becoming trapped. One type of an aortic dissection is a type A, which stands for a dissection that comprises the ascending aorta where emergency surgical intervention is required. Type B dissection usually arises in the descending aorta dissection allowing for medical management as the treatment of choice.
- Aortic aneurysms are another common problem that involves a weakening in the muscular walls of the part

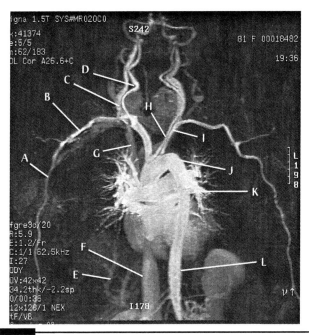

Figure 9-3 Chest vascular anatomy demonstrated in the coronal plane. This coronal acquisition of the vasculature of the chest was acquired with contrast-enhanced, 3D TOF MRA, which is the recommended technique for the evaluation of arterial structures of the chest. *A*, right brachial artery; *B*, right subclavian artery; *C*, right jugular vein; *D*, right vertebral artery; *E*, hepatic vessels; *F*, inferior vena cava; *G*, right subclavian vein; *H*, left common carotid artery; *I*, left subclavian artery; *J*, aortic arch; *K*, pulmonary vessels; *L*, thoracic aorta.

of the artery, which results in an enlargement of the damaged section. They can be caused by a congenital defect, a degenerative disease, or a syphilitic infection. Similar to aortic dissections, location of the aneurysm is important to determine the patient's course of treatment. A similar medical approach is used for treating aneurysms as with the dissections, thus aneurysms located in the ascending aorta or in the aortic arch are frequently treated surgically, and aneurysms in the descending aorta are treated medically.

- Early diagnosis is important for both aortic dissections and aneurysms resulting from complications that can occur with these conditions. If an aneurysm ruptures, massive bleeding can result in hypotension, coma, and death.
- Dissimilar to aneurysms, aortic stenosis is the narrowing of the aorta and occurs when two of the three flaps that comprise the aortic valve fuse together. This fusion narrows the opening to the aorta thus restricting blood flow out of the left ventricle into the aorta.
- Damage to the aortic valve can lead to aortic regurgitation, which occurs when some blood flows back into the left ventricle of the heart from the aorta after a heartbeat. Surgical intervention for repair or replacement of the valve is the necessary means for treatment.

Patient Positioning, Protocol, and Coil Selection for Magnetic Resonance Angiography of the Abdomen

Vascular imaging for each anatomic location within the body should be evaluated according to the vascular configuration, flow velocity, and vessel size.

- For the abdomen, arterial blood flow velocity is high, vessel diameter is large, and the flow is multidirectional. For this reason, 3-D, contrast-enhanced MRA is best to visualize abdominal vessels.
- To evaluate abdominal vessels, the coronal plane is the optimum.
- Patient positioning for MRA of the abdomen is generally similar to positioning for abdomen MRI. Patients are positioned supine in a torso-array coil or body coil and have MRI of the abdomen as well.
- Remember, patient screening is always recommended to avoid contraindications, and patients should always be provided hearing protection.

Abdomen Vascular Anatomy

Vascular anatomy of the abdomen can be evaluated by arterial and vascular structures.

Arteries of the Abdomen

- Defining the arterial system in the retroperitoneum involves the evaluation of the descending abdominal aorta, which is located anterior to the vertebral column (Figure 9-4).

- At the level of the first lumbar vertebrae (L1), the celiac axis arises anteriorly from the descending aorta and branches into the left gastric, hepatic, and splenic arteries.

- Following close to the celiac trunk inferiorly is the superior mesenteric artery (SMA), which also arises anteriorly from the descending aorta at the lower level of L1. The SMA branches to supply the small and large intestinal tracts.

- Both the right and left renal arteries lie inferior to the SMA and extend laterally from the descending aorta.

- Following along the abdominal aorta are the right and left gonadal arteries, which also extend laterally from the descending aorta and can be identified anterior to the psoas muscles that extend along the vertebral column.

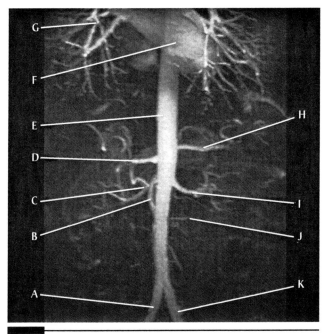

Figure 9-4 Abdomen vascular anatomy (arterial) is demonstrated in the coronal plane. This coronal acquisition of the vasculature of the abdomen was acquired with contrast-enhanced, 3D TOF MRA. *A*, right iliac artery; *B*, superior mesenteric artery (SMA); *C*, right renal artery; *D*, hepatic artery; *E*, abdominal aorta; *F*, heart; *G*, pulmonary vessels; *H*, splenic artery; *I*, left renal artery; *J*, spinal artery; *K*, left iliac artery.

Veins of the Abdomen

■ The inferior vena cava (IVC) is the first structure that needs to be identified in conjunction with the hepatic portal system. The IVC, which returns blood to the right atrium, lies slightly midline and anterior to the vertebral body.

■ Traveling inferiorly down the IVC are the three hepatic veins. The right and left hepatic veins extend laterally; the middle hepatic vein branches from the IVC anteriorly.

■ Next is the hepatic portal vein, which is located anterior to the IVC and posterior to both the duodenum and the head of the pancreas.

■ The left renal vein can be identified at the level of the second lumbar vertebrae (L2) as it crosses over the midline to drain its contents into the IVC. As it continues across the midline, the left renal vein can be seen anterior to the abdominal aorta and immediately inferior to the SMA.

■ Next is the splenic vein, which is located anterior to the left renal vein and follows midline to join the superior mesenteric vein to form the hepatic portal vein.

■ The inferior mesenteric vein empties into the splenic vein; both of these structures are located posterior to the pancreatic body.

Typical Vascular Abnormalities of the Abdomen

■ Renal artery stenosis and occlusions are often diagnosed with the use of MRA techniques.

■ Evaluation of the portal system is important since many disease processes can affect the vasculature system that is associated with the liver. Liver dysfunction is accompanied by diseases such as cirrhosis, hepatitis, carcinoma, and other related diseases.

■ Aortic dissection and aneurysm can also occur in the abdomen. For more information about these lesions, see the chest section.

Patient Positioning, Protocol, and Coil Selection for Magnetic Resonance Angiography of the Pelvis

Vascular imaging for each anatomic location within the body should be evaluated according to the vascular configuration, flow velocity, and vessel size.

- For the pelvis, arterial blood flow velocity is medium, vessel diameter is medium to small, and the flow is multidirectional. For this reason, 3-D, contrast-enhanced MRA is best to visualize pelvic vessels.
- To evaluate pelvic vessels, the sagittal plane is optimum.
- Patient positioning for MRA of the pelvis is generally similar to positioning for abdomen MRI. Patients are positioned supine in a torso-array coil or body coil. These patients have MRI of the pelvis along with the MRA study.
- Patient screening is always recommended to avoid contraindications, and patients should always be provided hearing protection.

Pelvic Vascular Anatomy

In the pelvis, the descending aorta branches into the common iliac arteries at the lower border of the fifth lumbar vertebrae (L5).

- Both the right and the left common iliac arteries divide into the external and internal iliac arteries.
- The external iliac arteries descend to form the femoral arteries that nourish the lower extremities.
- The internal iliac has many branches that supply blood to the pelvic wall and viscera.
- In the female pelvis, the anterior division of the internal iliac branches into the uterine artery, which supplies blood to the uterus.
- In the male pelvis, the pudendal artery arises from the anterior division of the internal iliac to supply blood to the penis.
- The posterior division of the internal iliac branches into the gluteal vessels in both the male and female pelvis.

Typical Vascular Abnormalities of the Pelvis

■ In the pelvis, assessment of the common iliac and femoral veins is important because the patient might undergo a surgical procedure. Frequently, clots can form after surgery and, when diagnosed early, further complications can be prevented.

■ Recently, MRI and MRA have been useful in evaluating the vasculature associated with the reproductive system. Impotence is the inability to maintain an erection because of an abnormality within the arterial or the venous system that supplies the blood to the penis.

■ Fibroids are a serious medical problem for many women. It has been documented that if the uterine artery is embolized, the collateral circulation will reconstitute the uterus, but the fibroid will die. For this reason, MRA of the female pelvis can be used to monitor such a treatment sequelae.

Patient Positioning, Protocol, and Coil Selection for Imaging the Extremities

Vascular imaging for each anatomic location within the body should be evaluated according to the vascular configuration, flow velocity, and vessel size.

■ For the peripheral vessels, arterial blood flow velocity is medium, vessel diameter is medium to small, and the flow is in one direction. For this reason, 2-D TOF may be acceptable for imaging the peripheral vessels, but with long imaging times.

■ To minimize scan times, 3-D, contrast-enhanced MRA with run-off may be optimal for the visualization of peripheral vessels.

■ To evaluate leg vessels, the coronal plane is optimal.

■ Patient positioning for MRA of the extremities is generally similar to positioning for coronal views of the extremities bilaterally. Patients are positioned in an extremity coil, torso-array coil, or body coil.

- For runoff MRA, a contrast agent is injected and imaging is acquired in three coronal steps: the lower abdomen and pelvis, femur and knees, and lower legs and possibly ankles.
- Patient screening is always recommended to avoid contraindications, and patients should always be provided hearing protection.

Extremity Vascular Anatomy

Vascular anatomy of the extremities begins at the aortic bifurcation in the abdomen.

- The aorta bifurcates into the right and left iliac arteries.
- The iliac arteries bifurcate into the internal (feeds the pelvis) and external iliac arteries.
- The external iliac artery continues to become the femoral artery.
- The femoral artery continues to the knee to become the popliteal artery.
- Below the knee, the popliteal trifurcates (trifurcation) into the anterior tibialis, posterior tibialis, and peroneal brevis.
- The anterior tibialis continues to become dorsalis pedis, the posterior tibialis continues to become the medial malleolus, and the peroneus brevis ends in the calf (Figure 9-5).

Typical Vascular Abnormalities of the Extremities

A number of typical abnormalities can be visualized by MRA and MRV of the extremities.

- Arterial abnormalities include vascular disease, plaque, or stenosis.
- Additional abnormalities include partial or complete occlusion or thrombosis.
- Venous vasculature of the extremities can also be evaluated for thrombosis or for evaluating potential grafts.

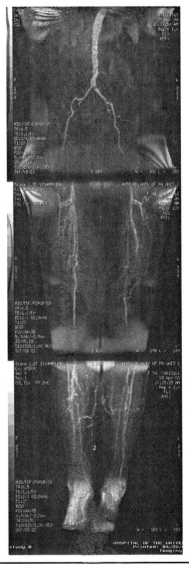

Figure 9-5 Vascular anatomy of the extremities demonstrates the coronal plane and was acquired with contrast-enhanced, 3D TOF MRA and a stepping table. The first step demonstrates the abdominal vessels, the second step the femoral vessels, and the third step the vessels of the lower leg.

REFERENCES

Applegate, E. *The sectional anatomy learning system*. Philadelphia: WB Saunders, 1991.

Barrafato D, Henkelman RM. Magnetic resonance imaging and surgical clips. *Can J Surg* 1984;27:509–512.

Bloem JL, Reiser MF, Vanel D. Magnetic resonance contrast agents in the evaluation of the musculoskeletal system. *Magn Reson Q* 1990;6:136–163.

Brasch RC, Weinmann HJ, Wesbey GE. Contrast-enhanced NMR imaging: animal studies using gadolinium-DTPA complex. *AJR* 1984;142:625–630.

Brasch RC. Introduction to the gadolinium class. *J Comput Assist Tomogr* 1993;17:S14–S18.

Brasch RC. New directions in the development of MR imaging contrast media. *Radiology* 1992;183:1–11.

Brasch RC. Rationale and applications for macromolecular Gd-based contrast agents. *J Magn Reson Med* 1991;22:282–287.

Brasch RC. Work in progress: methods of contrast enhancement for NMR imaging and potential applications. A subject review. *Radiology* 1983;147:781–788.

Brown JJ, Duncan JR, Heiken JP, et al. Perfluoroctylbromide as a gastrointestinal contrast agent for MR imaging: use with and without glucagon. *Radiology* 1991;181:455–460.

Brown MA, Carden JA, Coleman RE, et al. Magnetic field effects on surgical ligation clips. *J Magn Reson Imaging* 1987;5:443–453.

Chang CA, Sieving PF, Watson AD, Dewey TM. Ionic verses non-ionic MR imaging contrast media: operational definitions. *J Magn Reson Imaging* 1992;2:95–98.

Cooke P, Morris P. The effects of NMR exposure on living organisms. II. A genetic study of human lymphocytes. *Br J Radiol* 1981;54:622–625.

d'Agincourt L. MR contrast media open new avenues of diagnosis. *Diagn Imaging* 1988:82–90.

de Roos A, Doornbos J, Van der Wall EE, Van Voorthuisen AE. MR imaging of acute myocardial infarction; value of Gd-DTPA. *Am J Radiol* 1988;150:531–534.

Ebert M, Grossmann T, Heil W, et al. Nuclear magnetic resonance imaging with hyperpolarised helium-3. *Lancet* 1996;347:1297–1299.

Gaston A, Marsault C, Lacaze A, et al. External magnetic guidance of endovascular catheters with a superconducting magnet: preliminary trials. *J Neuroradiol* 1988;15:137–147.

Geard C, Osmak R, Hall E, et al. Magnetic resonance and ionizing radiation: a comparative evaluation in vitro of oncogenic and genotoxic potential. *Radiology* 1984;152:199–202.

Gibby WA. MR contrast agents; an overview. *Radiol Clin North Am* 1988;26:1047–1057.

Grady MS, Howard MA, Molloy JA, et al. Nonlinear magnetic stereotaxis: three dimensional in vivo remote magnetic manipulation of a small object in canine brain. *Med Phys* 1990;17:405–415.

Hamm B, Lanaido M, Saini S. Contrast enhanced magnetic resonance imaging of the abdomen and pelvis. *Magn Reson Q* 1990;6:108–135.

Heinrichs W, Fong P, Flannery M, et al. Midgestational exposure of pregnant balb/c mice to magnetic resonance imaging. *Magn Reson Imaging* 1988;6:305–313.

Heelan RT, Panicek DM, Burt ME, et al. Magnetic resonance imaging of the postpneumonectomy chest: normal and abnormal. *J Thorac Imaging* 1997;12:200–208.

Hesselink JR, Press GA. MR contrast enhancement of intracranial lesions with Gd-DTPA. *Radiol Clin North Am* 1988;26:873–886.

Kanal E, Gillen J, Evans J, et al. Survey of reproductive health among female MR workers. *Radiology* 1993;187:395–399.

Kauczor HU, Ebert M, Kreitner KF, et al. Imaging of the lungs using 3He MRI: preliminary clinical experience in 18 patients with and without lung disease. *J Magn Reson Imaging* 1997;7:538–543.

Kay H, Herkens R, Kay B. Effect of magnetic resonance imaging on Xenopus Laevis embryogenesis. *J Magn Reson Imaging* 1988;6:501–506.

Imakita S, Nishimura T, Yamada N, Naito H. Magnetic resonance imaging of cerebral infarction; time course of Gd-DTPA enhancement and CT comparison. *Neuroradiology* 1988;30:372–378.

Kuwatsuru R, Brasch RC, Muhler A, et al. Definition of liver tumors in the presence of diffuse liver disease: comparison of findings at MR imaging with positive and negative contrast agents. *Radiology* 1997;202:131–138.

Lauffer RB. Magnetic resonance contrast media; principles and progress. *Magn Reson Q* 1990;6(2):65–84.

Lenkinski RE. *MRI Contrast Agents.* MRI for Technologists Seminar Syllabus, 1990.

Lin W, Haacke EM, Smith AS, Clampitt ME. Gadolinium enhanced high resolution MR angiography with adaptive vessel tracking; preliminary results in the intracranial circulation. *J Magn Reson Imaging* 1992;2:277–284.

Lufkin RB. Magnetic resonance contrast mechanisms. In: Lufkin RB, ed. *The MRI Manual.* Chicago: Yearbook Publications, 1990.

Maravilla KR. Optimal use of MR agents; how much is enough? *AJNR* 1991; 12:881–883.

Merz CN, Berman DS. Imaging techniques for coronary artery disease: current status and future department of medicine. *Clin Cardiol* 1997;6:526–532.

McRobbie D, Foster M. Pulsed magnetic field exposure during pregnancy and implications for NMR fetal imaging: a study with mice. *J Magn Reson Imaging* 1985;3:231–234.

Nakamura T, Schorner W, Bittner RC, Felix R. The value of paramagnetic contrast agent gadolinium-DTPA in the diagnosis of pituitary adenomas. *Neuroradiology* 1988;30:481–486.

Ngo F, Blue J, Roberts W. The effect of a static magnetic field on DNA synthesis and survival of mammalian cells irradiated with fast neurons. *Magn Reson Med* 1987;5:307–317.

[No authors listed]. New developments in magnetic resonance contrast media. A global perspective on Gadoteriodol. Symposium proceedings, San Francisco, August 19, 1991. *Invest Radiol* 1992;27:575–577.

[No authors listed]. *Workshop on contrast-enhanced magnetic resonance syllabus.* SMRM Meeting May 23-25. Nappa, CA: 1991.

Peeling J, Lewis J, Samoiloff M, et al. Biological effects of magnetic fields: chronic exposure of the nematode Panagrellus Redivivus. *J Magn Reson Imaging* 1988;6:655–660.

Prasad N, Bushong S, Thronby J, et al. Effect of nuclear magnetic resonance on chromosomes of mouse bone marrow cells. *J Magn Reson Imaging* 1984; 2:37–39.

Prasad N, Wright D, Ford J, Thornby JI. Safety of 4-T MR imaging: study of effects on developing frog embryos. *Radiology* 1990;174:251–253.

Prasad N, Wright D, Forster J. Effect of nuclear magnetic resonance on early stages of amphibian development. *J Magn Reson Imaging* 1982;1:35–38.

Priatna A, Paschal CB, Shiavi RG. Evaluation of linear diaphragm-chest expansion models for magnetic resonance imaging motion artifact correction. *Comput Biol Med* 1999;2:111–127.

Ranney DF, Huffaker HH. Magnetic microspheres for the targeted controlled release of drugs and diagnostic agents. *Ann N Y Acad Sci* 1987:104–119.

Rubin DL, Muller HH, Nini-Murcia M, et al. Intraluminal contrast enhancement and MR visualization of the bowel wall: efficacy of PFOB. *J Magn Reson Imaging* 1991;1:371–380.

Schmiedl U, Moseley ME, Ogan MD, et al. Comparison of initial biodistribution patterns of Gd-DTPA and albumin-(Gd-DTPA) using rapid spin echo MR imaging. *J Comput Assist Tomogr* 1987;11:306–313.

Schmiedl U, Moseley MM, Ogan MD, et al. Contrast-enhancing Brasch RC. Inherent contrast in magnetic resonance imaging and the potential for contrast enhancement. The 1984 L. Henry Garland Lecture. *West J Med* 1985; 142:847–853.

Schwartz J, Crooks L. NMR imaging produces no observable mutations or cytotoxicity in mammalian cells. *AJR* 1982;139:583–585.

Shellock FG. *Guide to MR procedures and metallic objects: update 1999.* 5th ed. Philadelphia: Lippincott Williams & Wilkins Healthcare, 1999.

Shellock FG. MR imaging of metallic implants and materials: a compilation of the literature. *AJR* 1988;151:811–814.

Shellock FG, Crues JV. High-field strength MR imaging and metallic biomedical implants: an ex vivo evaluation of deflection forces. *AJR* 1988;151:389–392.

Shellock FG, Kanal E. *Magnetic resonance: bioeffects, safety, and patient management.* 2nd ed. New York: Lippincott-Raven Press, 1996.

Shellock FG, Kanal E. Policies, guidelines, and recommendations for MR imaging safety and patient management. *J Magn Reson Imaging* 1991;1:97–101.

Shellock FG, Morisoli S, Kanal E. MR procedures and biomedical implants, materials, and devices: 1993 update. *Radiology* 1993;189:587–599.

Shellock FG, Swengros-Curtis J. MR imaging and biomedical implants, materials, and devices: an updated review. *Radiology* 1991;180:541–550.

Sherry AD, Cacheris WP, Kuan KT. Stability constants for Gd3 + binding to model DTPA-conjugates and DTPA-proteins: implications for their use as magnetic resonance contrast agents. *Magn Reson Med* 1988;8:180–190.

Smith FW, MacLennan F. NMR imaging in human pregnancy: a preliminary study. *J Magn Reson Imaging* 1984;2:57–64.

Sze G. Gadolinium DTPA in spinal disease. *Radiol Clin North Am* 1988; 26:1009–1023.

Tyndall D, Sulik K. Effects of magnetic resonance imaging on eye development in the C57BL/6J mouse. *Teratology* 1991;43:263–275.

Wang SC, White DL, Pope JM, Brasch RC. Magnetic resonance imaging contrast enhancement versus tissue gadolinium concentration. *Invest Radiol* 1990; 25:S44–S45.

Weinmann HJ, Brasch RC, Press WR, Wesbey GE. Characteristics of gadolinium-DTPA complex: a potential NMR contrast agent. *AJR* 1984;142:619–624.

Wesbey GE, Engelstad BL, Brasch RC. Paramagnetic pharmaceuticals for magnetic resonance imaging. *Physiol Chem Phys Med NMR* 1984;16:145–155.

Westbrook C, Kaut C. *MRI in practice.* 2nd ed. Boston: Blackwell Science, 1994.

Wilcox A, Weinberg C, O'Connor J, et al. Incidence of early loss of pregnancy. *Physiol Chem Phys Med NMR* 1988;319:189–194.

Withers H, Mason K, Davis C. MR effect on murine spermatogenesis. *Radiology* 1985;156:741–742.

Wolf GL, Brady TJ. MR contrast agents enter growth phase. *J Magn Reson Imaging*

1991;1:2; Economic will dictate choice, not contrast safety or efficacy, *Magn Reson* 1991;1:30.

Wolff S, Crooks L, Brown P, et al. Test for DNA and chromosomal damage induced by nuclear magnetic resonance imaging. *Radiology* 1980;136:707–710.

Wolff S, James T, Young G, et al. Magnetic resonance imaging: absence of in vitro cytogenetic damage. *Radiology* 1985;155:163–165.

Yip YP, Capriotti C, Norbash SG, et al. Effects of MR exposure on cell proliferation and migration of chick motoneurons. *J Magn Reson Imaging* 1994;4:799–804.

Yip YP, Capriotti C, Talagala SL, Yip JW. Effects of MR exposure at 1.5 T on early embryonic development of the chick. *J Magn Reson Imaging* 1994;4:742–748.

Yip YP, Capriotti C, Yip JW. Effects of MR exposure on axonal outgrowth in the sympathetic nervous system of the chick. *J Magn Reson Imaging* 1995;4:457–462.

Young DB, Pawlak AM. An electromagnetically controllable heart valve suitable for chronic implantation. *ASAIO Trans* 1990;36:M421–M425.

Yousem DM, Ihmeidan I, Quencer R, Atlas SW. Paradoxically decreased signal intensity on post contrast short TR MR images. *AJNR* 1991;12:875–880.

Yousem DM, Patrone PM, Grossman RI. Leptomeningeal metastases; MR evaluation, *J Comput Assist Tomogr* 1990;14:255–261.

Yuh WTC, Engeleken JD, Muhonen MG, Mayr NA. Experience with high dose gadolinium MR imaging in the evaluation of brain metastases. *AJNR* 1992;13:335–345.

Yuh WTC, Fisher DJ, Engelken FD, Greene GM. MR evaluation of CNS tumors; dose comparison study with gadopentetate dimeglumine and gadoteridol. *Radiology* 1991;180:485–491.

Index